Surveillance Practices and Mental Health

This book examines how CCTV cameras expose the patient body inside the mental health ward, especially the relationship between staff and patients as surveillance subjects.

A key aspect of the book is that existing surveillance literature and mental health literature have largely ignored the influence of CCTV cameras on patient and staff experiences inside mental health wards. Research findings for this book suggest that camera use inside mental health wards is based on a perception of the violent nature of the mental health patient. This perception not only influences ethical mental health practice inside the ward but also impacts how patients experience the ward.

It is not known how and why CCTV camera use has expanded to its uses inside mental health wards. These include not only communal areas of the ward but also patient bedrooms. The research, therefore, examines how and why camera technology was introduced inside three Psychiatric Intensive Care Mental Health Units located in England, UK. Aimed at both undergraduate and postgraduate students, this book will appeal to sociology, mental health and surveillance studies students, as well as practitioners in mental health nursing, caseworkers and social caregivers.

Suki Desai has a background in social work and mental health. She has previously worked as a Mental Health Act commissioner and regional director for the Mental Health Act Commission. More recently, she has worked as a social work academic.

Routledge Studies in Surveillance

Kirstie Ball, William Webster, Charles Raab, Pete Fusey

Kirstie Ball is Professor in Management at University of St Andrews, UK

William Webster is Professor of Public Policy and Management at the University of Stirling, UK

Charles Raab is Professorial Fellow in Politics and International Relations at the University of Edinburgh, UK

Pete Fussey is a Professor in the Department of Sociology at University of Essex, UK

Surveillance is one of the fundamental sociotechnical processes underpinning the administration, governance and management of the modern world. It shapes how the world is experienced and enacted. The much-hyped growth in computing power and data analytics in public and private life, successive scandals concerning privacy breaches, national security and human rights have vastly increased its popularity as a research topic. The centrality of personal data collection to notions of equality, political participation and the emergence of surveillant authoritarian and post-authoritarian capitalisms, among other things, ensure that its popularity will endure within the scholarly community.

A collection of books focusing on surveillance studies, this series aims to help to overcome some of the disciplinary boundaries that surveillance scholars face by providing an informative and diverse range of books, with a variety of outputs that represent the breadth of discussions currently taking place. The series editors are directors of the Centre for Research into Information, Surveillance and Privacy (CRISP). CRISP is an interdisciplinary research centre whose work focuses on the political, legal, economic and social dimensions of the surveillance society.

Gender, Surveillance, and Literature in the Romantic Period
1780–1830
Lucy E. Thompson

For more information about this series, please visit: www.routledge.com/Routledge-Studies-in-Surveillance/book-series/RSSURV

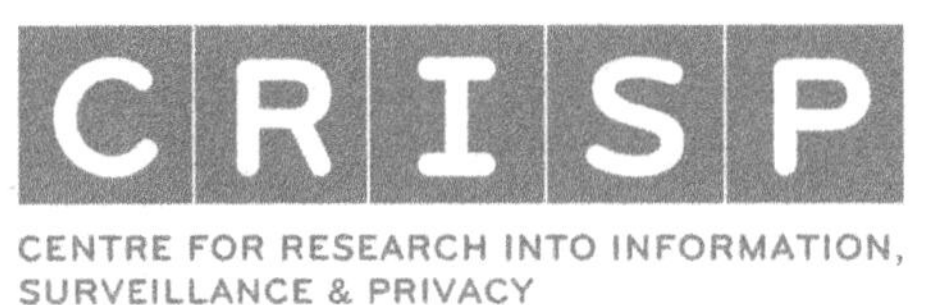

Surveillance Practices and Mental Health

The Impact of CCTV Inside Mental Health Wards

Suki Desai

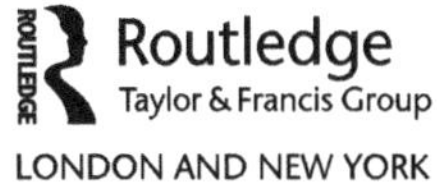

LONDON AND NEW YORK

First published 2022
by Routledge
2 Park Square, Milton Park, Abingdon, Oxon OX14 4RN

and by Routledge
605 Third Avenue, New York, NY 10158

Routledge is an imprint of the Taylor & Francis Group, an informa business

British Library Cataloguing-in-Publication Data
A catalogue record for this book is available from the British Library

Library of Congress Cataloging-in-Publication Data
Names: Desai, Suki, author.
Title: Surveillance practices and mental health: the impact of CCTV inside mental health wards / Suki Desai.
Description: Milton Park, Abingdon, Oxon ; New York, NY : Routledge, 2022. |
Series: Routledge studies in surveillance |
Includes bibliographical references and index.
Identifiers: LCCN 2021033893 (print) | LCCN 2021033894 (ebook) |
ISBN 9781032016085 (hardback) | ISBN 9781032016115 (paperback) |
ISBN 9781003179306 (ebook)
Subjects: LCSH: Psychiatry–Great Britain. |
Psychiatric hospital care–Great Britain–Case studies. |
Television in security systems. | Mental health services–Great Britain.
Classification: LCC RC450.G7 D47 2022 (print) |
LCC RC450.G7 (ebook) | DDC 362.2/10941–dc23
LC record available at https://lccn.loc.gov/2021033893
LC ebook record available at https://lccn.loc.gov/2021033894

ISBN: 978-1-032-01608-5 (hbk)
ISBN: 978-1-032-01611-5 (pbk)
ISBN: 978-1-003-17930-6 (ebk)

DOI: 10.4324/9781003179306

Typeset in Times New Roman
by Newgen Publishing UK

For my parents

Contents

Tables

Acknowledgements

My huge thanks to patients, staff and managers who contributed to this research. Your contributions were critical in shaping the analysis for this book. Thank you also to Mike McCahill for your support, critical comments and for constantly pushing me to improve my work. My thanks to Neil Thompson a long-time friend and a very accomplished social work author for your critical comments and support. Thank you to Routledge editorial team and Surveillance Studies Series editors for your comments and encouragement, especially Kirstie Ball and Lakshita Joshi. Finally, thank you Stuart for our journey and for all that is yet to come.

Chapter 1

Introduction

Surveillance practices and mental health

Background

This book is about how Closed-Circuit Television (CCTV) cameras or video surveillance cameras have infiltrated the mental health ward.[1] It examines how staff inside mental health wards make sense of camera technology and use it in their day-to-day activities. It also explores how patients as subjects of surveillance respond to camera monitoring inside the mental health ward. My interest in the growing use of CCTV cameras inside mental health wards came about during the time that I was appointed as a Mental Health Act commissioner and later as a regional director for the organization, the Mental Health Act Commission. The Mental Health Act Commission (now merged with the Care Quality Commission) was a National Health Service (NHS) special health authority. Its remit was to provide a safeguard for patients detained in hospital under the Mental Health Act 1983. This remit extended to England and Wales only as there are three distinct legal jurisdictions in relation to mental health law within the UK (England and Wales, Northern Ireland and Scotland). Mental Health Act commissioners visited hospitals to meet with those patients who are detained under the Mental Health Act 1983.

For me, the use of CCTV cameras inside the ward is linked to three main concerns. First of all, the issue around patient violence has increasingly been problematised within mental health literature and healthcare policy. Alongside this, and leading to the second concern, is the growing rights of staff not to be attacked by patients in their workplace. The third concern is how any response to resolving the issue of violence impacts on the patient experience inside the mental health ward. Prior to the deinstitutionalisation of patient care from asylums, asylum care was criticised for its segregation of patients from local communities and its security features. These security features included high walls and locked wards from which patients could not escape the hospital easily. Many of these security features have been adopted within modern mental health or post-institutional mental health hospitals.

DOI: 10.4324/9781003179306-1

Most modern mental health hospitals are not only difficult to leave, but they are also difficult to enter, and despite their reduced size and proximity to the community, they remain separate. In addition, the mixed model of mental healthcare provision including privately owned hospital care, independent or not-for-profit hospitals and NHS hospital care has meant that all mental health hospitals are more sensitive about their reputation and healthcare delivery. This also creates a tension between balancing the needs of patients, staff and the public where it is possible to lose sight of the patient who is at the receiving end of any changes to the ward environment.

During the time that I visited patients inside mental health hospitals as a commissioner and as a researcher, people often asked me whether I was for or against the cameras. Although I do not like the idea of having cameras inside my bedroom or living spaces, I can understand how the cameras can provide a feeling of safety inside mental health wards that feel unsafe. However, whether adding cameras into the ward environment is the solution is something that requires more debate. Through visiting and meeting with a range of patients and staff as a Mental Health Act commissioner, I was aware that the addition of cameras did change ward practices. This research was influenced by wanting to examine in what ways the cameras did or did not change the ward environment and the patient experience inside it. Therefore, the concluding chapter, Chapter 6, does not highlight a recommendation list of the benefits and limitations of camera use or how cameras should be used inside the ward. However, by drawing out key themes from the research data, my intention is that it will enable future managers, staff and patients to understand how placing cameras inside the mental health ward can influence mental health practice, including relationships between patients, staff and managers, and the cameras' impact on patients.

CCTV and the mental health hospital

The implementation and impact of electronic monitoring, especially CCTV cameras, have been extensively examined within social scientific literature. These investigations span its uses in public spaces and a range of other settings, including the commercial sector, housing estates, workplaces, schools and police cells (Marx, 1988; Davies, 1996; Norris et al., 1998; McCahill, 2002; Newburn and Hayman, 2002; Taylor, 2010). The use of CCTV surveillance has continued to expand in other areas including mental health wards. This book is based on research that recognises the social impact of camera use inside mental health wards. Mental health wards have certain identifiable features which make them different to other environments that use CCTV cameras inside them, for example:

- The majority of mental health wards are locked so that it is not easy for patients to walk out of them (CQC, 2018).

- Most patients inside mental health wards are likely to be detained under mental health legislation and are therefore inside the ward as involuntary patients (NHS Digital, October 2019).
- Those patients who are admitted inside them as voluntary patients fear that should they attempt to leave the mental health ward against the advice of their clinical team, they may be detained anyway. Under the Mental Health Act 1983 (in England and Wales, as amended in 2007), voluntary patients deemed unwell by staff and attempting to leave can be detained by them for up to 72 hours so that a formal assessment can take place (Sweeney et al., 2015).
- The average length of stay inside a mental health ward is 131.7 days. However, this average depends on the type of ward. For instance, the length of stay inside an acute ward is likely to be shorter than a rehabilitation ward (Samele and Urquía, 2015).
- The average length of stay inside a psychiatric intensive care unit (PICU) is 26.5 days. Most patients are discharged to acute mental health wards.

Although some wards have large spaces, not all places inside the ward can be accessed by patients, unless they are supervised by staff when they are using these spaces. Some of these places include the garden or courtyard areas, activity room and occupational therapy room. While staff can walk away from camera surveillance at the end of their shift, patients inside the ward are under continuous observation from cameras and therapeutic monitoring practices.

The use of surveillance technologies such as CCTV and body-worn cameras has been on the rise inside mental health wards since the early 1990s. Watching patients inside mental health hospitals is not a new activity. Cohen noted how patients were observed in solitary confinement for 24 hours inside Broadmoor Hospital so that "their 'true' psychiatric condition could surface and be observed" (1981 cited in Holyoake, 2013: 847). The potential benefits of CCTV surveillance can be extrapolated through hospital policies necessitating its implementation. However, what is less known about its use are the social consequences of such surveillance practices inside the ward. This is particularly relevant in how patients negotiate privacy and attempt to maintain their dignity when they are under constant observation, how they demonstrate individual autonomy, what is perceived as ethical watching and what is deemed as unethical watching inside the ward, how the filter of the cameras as a security feature affects watching, especially how nursing staff see patients (care vs. control), how the capacity of the cameras is limited through operationalisation by existing social relations between nursing staff and patients, political practice and cultural ward practices (McCahill, 2002), how CCTV monitoring converges with or undermines other practices and in what ways it creates equity inside the ward. These are some of the concerns that CCTV monitoring raises in the context of the mental health ward.

Coleman and McCahill (2012: 4) suggest that surveillance "is a matter of concern because it is never a neutral exercise". They identify a range of characteristics such as privacy, effectiveness, social order, equity and expansiveness of surveillance which they believe characterise the study of surveillance. In addition, other factors also need to be considered when examining surveillance practices inside mental health wards. For example, how surveillance technologies can compensate for any reduction in face-to-face relationships. Dix (2002) sums up several concerns related to the use of CCTV cameras inside mental health wards. These include intrusiveness, right to privacy and dignity, data protection, implications for nursing practices and the potential for negative effects on patients' mental state, especially where they are experiencing paranoia or delusions and generally questioning whether the cameras are in the patient's best interest. These concerns suggest that camera technology is not just about managing the safety of patients inside the ward or making the ward environment a secure place. The ability of the cameras to affect nursing practices and patient experience inside the ward suggests that the cameras' impact on staff and patients is much wider than their technological ability to manage ward security and safety. Therefore, the use of cameras in everyday practices inside the ward may influence what Moore (2011: 257) describes as the more "pastoral and productive" forms of surveillance that are already adopted inside the ward. These pastoral forms of surveillance are about positively engaging with patients in order to influence their behaviour.

CCTV and surveillance

Surveillance literature (discussed in more detail in Chapter 2) has also emphasised how CCTV cameras shape behaviour. Foucault's (1979) analysis of Bentham's Panopticon has been a central feature of how those people, who are subject to surveillance, modify their behaviour in line with the expectations of those people doing the watching. This expectation is founded on the assumption that the subjects of surveillance are rational, aware of their environment, understand the nature of technology by which they are being observed and can control their actions. These assumptions may not necessarily hold for mental health patients who are subject to a wide variety of cognitive distortions, perceptual limitations, emotional impairments and involuntary behaviours (Page, 2007). Therefore, patients with mental health conditions are different in that the nature of their condition may impact their perception and experience of CCTV cameras differently from those people who are fully aware of how such technology can influence their behaviour. For example, for some mental health conditions, the feelings of paranoia may become heightened for patients, where they believe that the cameras have some special significance to them, resulting in the cameras creating more distress and possibly inciting disturbing behaviour, which is the opposite of their function.

CCTV surveillance is all-encompassing. Cameras do not just watch patients; they also watch staff and any other person coming into the ward environment, including the patients' family and friends. Therefore, cameras also broaden out the scope of surveillance beyond the patient. It can be argued that the widening of surveillance in this way can also benefit patients. For example, the families of Esmin Green in the United States and Wang Xiuying in China placed CCTV grabs on the World Wide Web to draw attention and seek justice for the neglect and abuse experienced by these patients from those people tasked to look after them (Desai, 2010). Without CCTV footage, it would have been difficult for them to prove that neglect and abuse may have been contributory factors in their deaths. In this way, surveillance practices are not limited to hierarchical watching and accountability. The appeal of the cameras inside the ward for patients and staff is that they provide the possibility of equity inside it, where the cameras have the potential to prove to others that they were victims of violence, theft or unwanted attention. However, camera evidence is not value-free and has ethical implications for patients as well as staff and managers. For example, although the cameras do show body movements, these movements are not linked to one narrative. Each narrative, whether it is staff or patient narrative, is open to a range of possibilities about what happened in a given situation. Also, the fact that the ward is governed by rules, legislation and institutionalised practices that promote a hierarchical structure suggests that patient and staff narratives may not have the same authority. This perspective suggests that CCTV surveillance inside the ward could be limited to one-way viewing where patients in particular have little control about how they are seen and what is seen. The research for this book therefore also opens up surveillance to examine how patients as subjects of surveillance use cameras to manage how they are seen and what is seen (see Chapter 5).

Camera technology, whether this is CCTV or body-worn cameras, exposes behaviour. It is this aspect of the technology which makes them appealing, even though there is no clear evidence of their ability to bring any order inside the ward. They are perceived as enabling tools because they are thought to protect patient and staff equally. They are believed to create a secure ward environment because it is assumed that patients and staff know that they are being watched. They allow patients and staff to move around in tight ward spaces because should anything go wrong, they can expose any anomalies within patient and staff narratives. They are perceived as bringing justice to patients and staff who are attacked by other patients. They are also seen as helpful in improving the ward environment by exposing weak points in the ward where patients can escape or strangers can get inside it. Their ability to expand surveillance inside the ward means that they also have the ability to improve nursing care by exposing poor and unsafe practices. In these ways, their uses are deemed to be endless because their full potential inside the ward remains unknown. In reality, the cameras do more than keep staff and patients safe inside the ward, they also serve a purpose for a whole range of agendas of which some are linked to safety and security of the physical environment of the ward and others that are about exposing poor nursing care or medical care, staff management, resolving potential litigation disputes and other wider political agendas related to mental health care.

Lyon (2001) has argued that caring surveillance has been unjustly neglected by social researchers. Clinical input inside the ward is not only about medicating the patient. Patients who have lost control of their behaviour as a result of their mental health condition also have to learn to manage their behaviour in ways that are acceptable to society. An inability to do so means that the patient cannot be discharged from the hospital until this is the case. Behavioural responses used inside mental health wards are reliant on engineering patient responses by modifying those behaviours that are not perceived as helpful to them. To do this, the mental health ward adopts a combination of tough responses (sometimes experienced as punitive by patients) and inducements (such as having time off the ward). This general function of the ward has not radically changed since providing mental health care inside asylums where staff have responsibility for the day-to-day management of patient behaviour and the overall responsibility of patient care lies with the patient's consultant psychiatrist. The role of the consultant psychiatrist in the context of the ward has received little attention. Their removal from the everyday management of the patient places them in a unique position as an arbitrator. They are the ones that staff appeal to when a patient is difficult to control. They are also the ones that patients count as important in the ward because they hold the power to decide whether the patient needs to continue to stay in the ward or is ready for discharge. The hierarchical nature of the ward is therefore also apparent in the position of the patient's consultant psychiatrist. Surveillance inside the mental health ward, therefore, is not limited to techniques of surveillance or technologies of surveillance (such as CCTV, or body-worn cameras, or nurse monitoring practices). It also encompasses positional power located in the body of the consultant psychiatrist. This surveillance is different because it does not solely rely on behavioural or other techniques; it is based on pastoral care which encompasses the need to guide, heal and sustain the patient based on the authority and wisdom embodied in the representation of the consultant psychiatrist (Foucault, 2009).

This aspect of pastoral care is significant to surveillance practices inside the ward because it also influences how patient behaviour is shaped. Therefore, as Moore (2011: 257) has argued, surveillance practices inside the ward are not necessarily technocratic, but they can also be "intimate, pastoral and productive". She suggests that benevolence and coercion are inextricably linked. Lianos (2003: 415) concurs with this view suggesting that "institutional control is often perceived as beneficial and sometimes even liberating". For some patients, the mental health hospital is not a negative experience, including for those patients who are detained under mental health legislation. These patients welcome the feeling of safety of the mental health ward and the ability to gain control over their mental health condition. However, Moore's (2011) analysis of therapeutic surveillance is also built on personal knowledge and relationship with the person who is watched. Therefore, how the cameras influence how knowledge about each patient is gathered, and the possible reduction or loss of face-to-face contact between staff and patient, also raises concerns about how care and control are balanced inside the ward.

Finally, there are several therapeutic practices adopted inside modern mental health hospitals, especially in the management of aggressive patient behaviour, which are not dissimilar to those practices carried out inside asylums. These include the use of forced medication to sedate patients, usually given intramuscularly and referred to by patients as "the injection", use of additional prescribed medication to calm patients down, use of seclusion where the patient is segregated from other patients and the use of full-body restraint, where the patient is held down by several staff. These ways of controlling or managing patient behaviour are perceived as coercive methods of intervention where the patient has little choice in what is done to them. Newer technologies such as CCTV cameras and body-worn cameras not only allow the modern mental health ward to stand apart from asylums, they are also perceived as new ways of controlling and managing aggressive patient behaviour. However, the introduction of cameras into the ward environment has assumed that the cameras do not influence staff and patient relationships and that the widening of surveillance is a good thing. Therefore, less emphasis has been placed on how the cameras influence or change existing nursing practices inside the mental health ward.

Surveillance literature suggests that CCTV cameras not only have the potential to change behaviour, but they can also influence how people are seen. The two-dimensional viewing of people through CCTV monitors changes what is looked at and what is seen (Koskela, 2000). Also, those people under surveillance do not passively accept it and often find ways to resist it (Walsh, 2018). While surveillance literature has examined the social impact of CCTV cameras in the context of open-street surveillance or its influence inside shopping centres and workplaces, very little has been said about its social impact inside mental health wards. Mental health wards provide a unique surveillance space because the cameras not only watch staff, they also watch patients and visitors to the ward. It is a restricted space where patients and, to some extent, staff are confined inside locked spaces. Whereas managers are interested in staff behaviour, staff are interested in patient behaviours. Also, whereas staff can understand why the cameras are in the ward and adjust their behaviour accordingly, patients often do not always understand why the cameras are in the ward because of their mental health condition. These influences create a complex network of concerns that have the potential to undermine pastoral and ethical care.

Methodology

The methodology used in the fieldwork for the research was ethnography. According to Atkinson and Hammersley (1998: 110), the benefits of adopting ethnography as a methodology are that it:

- Allows the researcher to explore the nature of a particular social phenomenon (for example, CCTV inside a mental health ward) without testing out a particular hypothesis.
- Enables the researcher to work with unstructured data.
- Allows the investigation of a small number of studies in depth.
- Allows an analysis of data that involves interpretation of a phenomenon.

Higginbottom et al. (2013: 1) emphasise that ethnography involves the describing of a culture that includes a "process of learning about people by learning from them". Furthermore, they claim that ethnography has the potential to link micro and macro concerns. Therefore, they believe that ethnography can link everyday interactions within the context in which they occur, making it a valuable tool for researching healthcare concerns. These concerns, they claim, include not only those dimensions of a culture that are known but also the "covert or tacit dimensions", which may not be voiced by members of a particular culture but are still shared by them (Higginbottom et al., 2013: 1). The ideal way in which to learn about others is, according to Van Maanen (1988), through living with and living like those they are studying. However, what this means in practice can be difficult to quantify. In the context of this research, the use of ethnography as a methodology is perceived as a blending of science and art, where coding was used to manage emerging data. It was perceived as an appropriate methodology, as it allowed the researcher to be embedded in the ward environment in order to understand the patient's lived experience of the cameras.

Knoblauch (cited in Kühn, 2013) highlights the developing nature of ethnography as a research methodology and its use in a range of disciplines. He uses the term "focused ethnography" to differentiate between one of the newer forms of ethnographic practice from the more traditional anthropological forms. The use of focused ethnography, as described by Knoblauch (2005), is a relatively well-recognised methodology within health research. On a pragmatic level when applying for NHS ethics approval and seeking access to research sites through NHS research and development departments, it has been beneficial to use terminology that is familiar to the field. However, focused ethnography was also considered relevant for this research for other reasons. For example, as Kühn (2013) explains, within focused ethnography, field stays are shorter because specific aspects of the field are studied with a purpose as opposed to the whole field. This research aimed to identify and understand the phenomena of CCTV and how it impacts patients and staff inside the mental health ward. The construction of knowledge repertoires is, therefore, based around how the cameras shape patient and staff behaviour and how they cohere (or not) with other practices inside the ward as well as the ethical concerns that they raise.

Wall (2015: 8) also suggests that within focused ethnographic research, participants may not necessarily know one another, and therefore the researcher focuses on their "common behaviours and shared experiences" while working from the assumption that they share a cultural perspective. All three wards were PICUs, which meant that they shared some similar features. For example, the average length of stay in PICU wards is much shorter than that inside other mental health wards, such as an acute ward. Inside PICUs, once patients are deemed not to require intensive care, they are occasionally discharged from the ward or more likely transferred to other wards. This meant that the turnover of patients inside each ward was much higher, and this also limited patient's ability to get to know one another. Patients in all three PICUs were detained under mental health legislation, and this meant that there were restrictions on their movements and ability to access some parts of the ward, including their ability to leave the ward. Patients in all three wards were subject to nurse observation practices, and while each ward had certain practices around mealtimes, visiting times and items that patients could bring into the ward, all patients were restricted to what they could do. Staff in all three wards were also typified by a core team of staff and a whole range of agency and bank staff, who were employed to cover shifts when there were not enough staff in the ward. This practice was quite common, and therefore it was also the case that not all staff knew one another on every shift.

My entry into fieldwork was marked by the fact that I entered it with specific intent. This was to examine how camera use impacted patients and staff inside the ward. Also, I had prior knowledge of the field in relation to professional work experience. I was interested in how macro analysis and perception of CCTV cameras, such as "Big Brother" watching, linked to their everyday uses inside the ward. This familiarity with the ward environment and the intention of entering the field with a specific goal meant that I was not entering the ward as a traditional ethnographic researcher. As Wall (2015: 15) states, most ethnographers do not enter the field with a specific research question, and they often "begin the project with no prior conceptions". My previous knowledge about the ward environment was also the driving factor in what I wanted to know. It was this knowledge that led me to want to know more about the cameras, for instance, whether patients and staff knew about CCTV use inside the ward, why they believed the cameras were inside the ward, what information they had been given about the cameras, how they experienced the cameras and how they reacted to being watched by the cameras. These questions arose during the time that I was employed as a commissioner and regional director with the Mental Health Act Commission. I was also aware that some patients welcomed having cameras inside the ward and others did not. It was therefore difficult to form an opinion as to how they benefitted patients.

The methods used to gain a better understanding of the cameras inside the ward included an examination of documentary evidence, ethnographic observations and qualitative semi-structured interviews with patients, staff and managers. The research period was from May 2017 to February 2018. A total of 198 hours of fieldwork observations were undertaken across three PICUs. Access inside each PICU was for two hours a day. Observations took place at different times of the day and night time, including weekdays and weekends. All three PICUs were NHS Foundation Trust organisations. PICUs were not specifically targeted. Access was negotiated with managers who were interested in knowing how CCTV affects patients and staff inside the wards. The organisation National Association of Psychiatric Intensive Care and Low Secure Units (NAPICU) was also very supportive in enabling access and taking an interest in the research. Without the support of NAPICU and the NHS, it would have been difficult to do this research.

In total, 14 patients, 27 staff and 10 managers were interviewed. Patient interviews, P1 to P14, included 4 females and 10 males. Staff interviews, S1 to S27, included 18 females and 9 males. Manager interviews, M1 to M10, included four females and six males. Staff interviews included mental health nurses and healthcare workers who either were employed permanently by the Trust or were agency and bank staff who covered a shift on a temporary basis. Agency staff were generally employed by a private agency, and bank staff were staff employed by the Trust. Manager interviews included ward managers, managers responsible for hospital and PICU security and senior managers responsible for the overall management of the PICU.

The original aim of the research was also to examine documentation in the form of minutes from meetings where it was assumed that discussion about camera implementation inside the ward was held. However, in reality, this level of documentary evidence was not available. Managers could not locate it, or there was no recorded discussion. Therefore, this research has predominantly drawn on the advice provided by NAPICU in their various documents discussed in more detail in Chapter 4. Two of the three PICUs involved in the research had minimal standard operational procedures in the use of bedroom cameras and cameras inside seclusion. None of the three units had any procedures relating to the use of cameras in communal area.

To research the three PICUs, an application for ethics approval was also made to the NHS Research Ethics Committee. Ethics approval was also sought to carry out intrusive research under the Mental Capacity Act 2005. Therefore, those patients who either permanently or temporarily lack the capacity to make decisions themselves, including deciding whether they want to be included in the research or not, could be included in the research. This additional ethical approval was sought in order to include observation of patients inside the ward and observation of patients in seclusion who may not have the capacity to understand the nature of the research. Ethics approval for the research was granted without any additional amendments to the research protocol.

Chapters

The core analysis underpinning this book is based on the following findings from the research:

1 The introduction of CCTV cameras inside the ward is driven by a lack of clear focus and operational procedures in their use.
2 The implementation of CCTV cameras inside mental health wards is based on a perception of the violent nature of the mental health patient.
3 That camera use has ethical implications for mental health practices inside the ward.
4 The cameras' effect on patients as surveillance subjects does alter their experience of the mental health ward.
5 That patients adopt a range of strategies to undermine CCTV surveillance.
6 That existing literature has underplayed the impact of CCTV surveillance on patients who are already exposed to a range of surveillance practices inside the mental health ward.

These and other aspects are developed more fully in the following chapters:

Chapter 2: Theory: Surveillance practices inside mental health hospitals

In this chapter, I explore how surveillance practices related to patient care inside the mental health hospital has been influenced by panoptic theoretical inquiry, based on Foucauldian analysis of Bentham's Panopticon. The chapter sets out how power inside the mental health ward functions to shape patient behaviour. Although Foucault (2008) describes the mental health hospital as a panoptic curing machine, there is very little literature on how the mental health hospital is or continues to remain so. This chapter suggests that it is Foucault's analysis of sovereign power, panoptic power and pastoral power that is central to the production of disciplinary behaviour. By raising the potential for new surveillance technologies to cohere to existing uncertainties and wider political agendas related to mental health care, the chapter also draws on post-Panoptic approaches to examine how CCTV cameras have the potential to cohere to these wider agendas inside the ward. Finally, the chapter also examines how people, as subjects of CCTV surveillance, resist camera surveillance.

Chapter 3: Implementing CCTV cameras inside mental health wards

This is the first of the three chapters which presents empirical data from the research. In this chapter, I aim to examine how the cameras, initially used to manage security within the periphery of the hospital, have managed to find their way inside the ward. The chapter highlights manager's decision-making when considering using cameras inside the ward. This includes aspects around managing safety, maintaining a secure ward environment, allowing patients to have choices and aiming to create litigation-free ward spaces and practices. The chapter draws attention to the fact that unlike other equipment and fixtures inside mental health wards, CCTV cameras have received less attention. The chapter also describes the three research sites and the placement of cameras within each site. It examines the various uses of cameras inside the ward, for example, inside patient bedrooms, the decision to implement live-feed cameras only, the decision to use recording facilities and how the placement of cameras impacted privacy for staff and patients inside the ward. These, together with other factors related to camera use inside wards, are discussed alongside manager's reflections on what they wanted the cameras to achieve.

Chapter 4: Practice implications and CCTV surveillance

In this chapter, I set out how staff used CCTV cameras as part of their day-to-day activities inside the ward. There is currently very little national policy or advice on the use of cameras inside mental health wards. The chapter, therefore, draws on the guidance adopted by NAPICU to examine a range of beneficial uses of CCTV identified by them (NAPICU, 2014; NAPICU and NHS Clinical Commissioners, 2016). These and other uses of the cameras are discussed in the context of how they influence social and therapeutic relationships between staff and patients.

Chapter 5: Patient and staff experiences of CCTV

In this final of the three empirical data chapters, I highlight patient and staff experience of being surveilled by CCTV cameras. By exposing the surveillance subject that is produced as a result of CCTV surveillance, the data presented in this chapter is divided into four broad sections. The first and second parts include patient and staff awareness of cameras and how they felt about the cameras, including why they believed the cameras were inside the ward. The third and fourth parts are linked to patient responses and attempts to resist camera surveillance. Responses to surveillance were initially observed by Scott (1985) who claimed that small-scale and individual everyday protests had been largely ignored by ethnographers and social scientists. Foucault has also argued that power and resistance involves a complex interplay of power that is not necessarily about collective action but is based on individualised actions (Foucault cited in Johansson and Vinthagen, 2014). The chapter, therefore, examines how patients attempted to neutralise CCTV surveillance inside the ward.

Chapter 6: Conclusion: The politics of surveillance and mental health

This final chapter is divided into two parts. The first part examines how undertaking research inside mental health wards has contributed to the current theoretical debate in the sociological understanding of CCTV cameras. The second part examines the use of CCTV cameras inside mental health wards and the social implications of this on the patient experience. Three themes are picked up concerning implications for practice. These include the negative categorisation of patients through the criminalisation of their behaviour at a time when they are most vulnerable, the creation of safeguarding concerns as a result of the exposure of women's bodies and the undermining of ethical mental health practice.

Note

1 The term CCTV is predominantly used throughout this book to distinguish the use of Closed-Circuit Television cameras from other camera uses inside the mental health ward such as body-worn cameras.

Bibliography

Atkinson, P. and Hammersley, M. (1998). "Ethnography and participant observation," in N.K. Denzin and Y.S. Lincoln (eds), *Strategies of Qualitative Inquiry*, London: Sage, pp. 110–136.

Care Quality Commission (CQC). (2018). *The Stare of Care in Mental Health Services 2014–2017: Findings from CQC's Programme of Comprehensive Inspections of Specialist Mental Health Services*, Care Quality Commission, Gallowgate, Newcastle-upon-Tyne, England.

Coleman, R. and McCahill, M. (2011). *Surveillance and Crime*, London: Sage.

Davies, S. (1996). *Big Brother: Britain's Web of Surveillance and the New Technological Order*, London: Pan Books.

Deleuze, G. (1992). "Postscript on the societies of control," *October*, 59: 3–7.

Desai, S. (2010). "Violence and surveillance: Some unintended consequences of CCTV monitoring within mental health hospital wards," *Surveillance and Society*, 8(1): 85–92.

Dix, R. (2002). "Observation and technology: Logical progression or ethical nightmare," *National Association of Psychiatric Intensive Care Units Bulletin*, 2(4): 21–29.

Foucault, M. (1979). *Discipline and Punish: The Birth of the Prison*, New York: Vintage.

Foucault, M. (2008). *Psychiatric Power: Lectures at the Collège de France 1973–1974*, edited by Jacques Lagrange and translated by Graham Burchell, Basingstoke: Palgrave.

Foucault, M. (2009). *Security, Territory, Population: Lectures at the Collège de France 1977–1978*, edited by Michel Senellart and translated by Graham Burchell, Basingstoke: Palgrave.

Higginbottom, G.M.A., Pillay, J.J. and Boadu, N.Y. (2013). "Guidance on performing focused ethnographies with an emphasis on healthcare," *The Qualitative Report*, 18(17): 1–6.

Holyoake, D.-D. (2013). "I spy with my little eye something beginning with O: Looking at what the myth of 'doing observations' means in mental health nursing culture," *Journal of Psychiatric and Mental Health Nursing*, 20: 840–850.

Johansson, A. and Vinthagen, S. (2014). "Dimensions of everyday resistance: An analytical framework," *Critical Sociology*, 42(3): 417–435.

Knoblauch, H. (2005). "Focused ethnography," *Forum Qualitative Sozialforschung / Forum: Qualitative Social Research*, 6(3): Art. 44. Available online: http://nbn-resolving.de/urn:nbn:de:0114-fqs0503440 [accessed 11 April 2016].

Koskela, H. (2000). "The gaze without eyes: Video-surveillance and the changing nature of urban space," *Progress in Human Geography*, 24(2): 243–265.

Kühn, J.-M. (2013). "Focused ethnography as research method: A case study of techno music producers in home recording studios," *Dancecult: Journal of Electronic Dance Music Culture*, 5(1). Available online: https://dj.dancecult.net/index.php/dancecult/article/view/356/361 [accessed 11 April 2016].

Lianos, M. (2003). "Social control after Foucault," *Surveillance and Society*, 1(3): 412–430.

Lyon, D. (2001). *Surveillance and Society: Monitoring Everyday Life*, Buckingham: Open University Press.

Marx, G.T. (1988). *Undercover: Police Surveillance in America*, Berkley: University of California.

McCahill, M. (2002). *The Surveillance Web: The Rise of the Visual Surveillance in an English City*, Cullompton: Willan Publishing.

Moore, D. (2011). "The benevolent watch: Therapeutic surveillance in drug treatment court," *Theoretical Criminology*, 15(3): 255–268.

National Association of Psychiatric Intensive Care and Low Secure Units (NAPICU). (2014). *National Minimum Standards for Psychiatric Intensive Care in General Adult Services*, East Kilbride: NAPICU International Press.

National Association of Psychiatric Intensive Care and Low Secure Units (NAPICU) and NHS Clinical Commissioners. (2016). *Guidance for Commissioners of Psychiatric Intensive Care Units (PICU)*, East Kilbride: NAPICU International Press.

National Health Service (NHS) Digital. (October 2019). *Mental Health Act Statistics, Annual Figures 2018–2019*. Available online: http://digital.nhs.uk [accessed 14 January 2021].

Newburn, T. and Hayman, S. (2002). *Policing, Surveillance and Social Control*, Cullompton: Willan Publishing.

Norris, C., Moran, J. and Armstrong, G. (1998). *Surveillance, Closed Circuit Television and Social Control*, Aldershot: Ashgate.

Page, M. (2007). "Engaging the disengaged: Collecting the views of patients in low secure unit on methods of observation," *Journal of Psychiatric Intensive Care*, 3(1): 13–19.

Samele, C. and Urquía, N. (2015). "Editorial: Psychiatric inpatient care: Where do we go from here?" *Epidemiology and Psychiatric Sciences*, 24: 371–375.

Scott, J.C. (1985). *Weapons of the Weak: Everyday Form of Peasant Resistance*, New Haven: Yale University Press.

Sweeney, A., Gillard, S., Wykes, T. and Rose, D. (2015). "The role of fear in mental health service users' experiences: A qualitative exploration," *Social Psychiatry and Psychiatric Epidemiology*, 50(7): 1079–1087.

Taylor, E. (2010). "I spy with my little eye: The use of CCTV in schools and the impact of privacy," *Sociological Review*, 58(3): 381–405.

Van Maanen, J. (1988). *Tales of the Field: On Writing Ethnography*, 2nd edition, Chicago: The University of Chicago Press.

Wall, S. (2015). "Focused ethnography: A methodological adaptation for social research in emerging contexts," *Forum Qualitative Sozialforschung / Forum: Qualitative Social Research*, 16: 1. Available online: www.qualitative-research.net/index.php/fqs/article/view/2182/3728 [accessed 15 March 2015].

Walsh, J.P. (2018). "Countersurveillance," in M. Deflem (ed), *The Handbook of Social Control*, Chichester: Wiley Blackwell, pp. 374–389.

Chapter 2

Theory

Surveillance practices inside mental health hospitals

Introduction

This chapter suggests that it is not necessarily vast changes in healthcare practices that make the modern mental hospital stand apart from the asylum but how power is used inside wards to change or influence patient behaviour. The concept of power has typically been distilled into the powerful and the powerless or hierarchical power. For example, one of the appeals of the novel and film *One Flew Over the Cuckoo's Nest* is the antagonistic and nasty character of nurse Ratched who, in her responses to patients, provides a clear distinction between the underdog patient and the evil nurse (Kesey, 1973). Kesey's novel draws clear power delineation between patients and staff, between staff and orderlies and between staff and the consultant psychiatrist. Power is ordered hierarchically, and this hierarchy can be seen. Inside modern mental health hospitals, power is more fragmented and therefore is not as easily distinguished. For example, the consultant psychiatrist who has the power to discharge a detained patient from the ward is not located inside it. It is not always easy to know who the ward staff are as nursing staff do not always wear uniforms. In addition, the ward often has bank and agency staff who may or may not know patients and usually perform different tasks to permanent ward staff. Although the smooth running of the ward is the responsibility of the ward manager, on a day-to-day basis, the ward is overseen by the nurse in charge. Therefore, it is not always easy to understand hierarchical power structures inside them. This makes power in the context of the modern mental health ward much more ubiquitous. When patients want to complain about their detention, they really want their consultant psychiatrist to do something about this. However, these matters are dealt with by managers who may also not be located inside the ward. It therefore becomes difficult for patients to decipher who to appeal to when they are unhappy about their detention or their care inside the ward, even though patients have more rights (in comparison to asylum care) and there are several mechanisms by which patients can make a complaint and make an appeal about their detention and other matters that concern them. Patient care suggests that they

DOI: 10.4324/9781003179306-2

have a say or a voice inside the ward about their mental health care and yet mental health literature suggests that they remain powerless in changing their experience (Gilburt et al., 2008; Lilja and Hellzén, 2008; Edal et al., 2019). To understand how power is used inside the ward to make patients the subject of surveillance, this chapter examines Foucault's analysis of sovereign power, disciplinary power and pastoral power, to explore how these forms of power influence mental healthcare practices inside the ward (Foucault, 1979, 2009).

Background

There are several interpretations of how people with mental health conditions became confined. Porter (2002) and Scull (1993) provide a useful chronological account of the confinement of madness and the rise of asylums in the care and treatment of madness as a disease. Foucault (1971) places less emphasis on this and instead has based his interpretation on the notion that normality can only be achieved by suppression and exclusion of the abnormal within modern society. He believed that it is not madness that drives how society perceives it, but the society in which madness exists. Therefore, how madness changes, is dependent on how each society has treated it. For Foucault, each historical period has treated madness differently, and the only stable entity is the split between madness and reason (Foucault, 1971). Hence, what is classed as madness and unreasonable behaviour in the past is not the same as what is perceived as unreasonable behaviour today. For example, openly practising homosexuality, or admitting to being gay or lesbian, having children out of wedlock and remaining unmarried for a woman were perceived as unreasonable behaviours some 70 years or so ago, which in themselves were sometimes reasons to confine people inside asylums. These behaviours are largely accepted today, and some behaviours such as having children out of wedlock are perceived as normal. While people might contest this notion or believe it to be the case, what remains the same is that the confinement of madness is done to change or normalise what society perceives as unreasonable behaviour.

The normalisation of behaviour is dependent upon watching and observing patients. Inside the mental health ward, this is not just about controlling patient behaviours and urges, it is also about treating the patient so that they can lead a fulfilled and normal life away from the hospital. Observation and noting changes in patient behaviour is a critical foundation of the mental health ward, and therefore it is not surprising that CCTV technology has found its way inside it because it opens up new ways of observing patients. CCTV cameras are not only associated with observing or looking at people. The observation or watching of people is undertaken with an intention, whether that is to catch them in the act of wrongdoing, to reprimand them or to influence their behaviour in other ways. Mental health literature has largely tended to ignore any theoretical analysis of CCTV technology inside mental health wards. However, this literature has been critical of monitoring practices inside the ward (Gastaldo and Holmes, 1999; Stevenson and Cutcliffe, 2006; Springer, 2015). This includes drawing on Foucault's analysis of panoptic power in the critique of nurse observation practices (Holmes, 2001).

The mental health ward is not only defined by nurse observation practices. It also uses a combination of other techniques, including the use of segregating a patient by placing them in seclusion from other patients, the use of forced medication (or the "injection") and the use of full-body restraint, where several staff hold the patient down on the ground or their bed until they have calmed down. These practices like nurse observations have also been passed down from asylum care. These latter forms of controlling patient behaviours are about applying physical force on the patient body and are synonymous with what Foucault (1979) refers to as sovereign power. Some mental health wards have chosen to move away from these practices. Of the three research sites, one site did not have any seclusion facilities within it which meant that patients could not be easily segregated from other patients and their behaviour had to be managed in other ways. Unlike sovereign power based on the physical control of the body, CCTV cameras are associated with panoptic power. Panoptic power is not about the visibility of power, it is about the invisibility of power and not knowing who is watching your behaviour, when they are watching and, most importantly, in the context of the mental health ward, what judgements they are making about your behaviour. The control of power inside the ward and in what measures the patient body is regulated is, according to Foucault (2008), reliant on pastoral power and the scrutinising of the patient body through medical examination undertaken by the patient's consultant psychiatrist. The understanding of a patient's behaviour, therefore, is not solely determined by one dominant form of power. It relies on the administration of tough responses (which can include "the injection" or full-body restraint), showing kindness, empathy and respect (which can include giving patient's concessions like having time off the ward, having visitors) and the expertise of the medical examination conducted by the consultant psychiatrist. It is the careful integration of these techniques based on healthcare and surveillance practices, which includes sovereign, panoptic and pastoral power that is used to manage or discipline patient behaviour. As a surveillance tool, CCTV cameras can affect the nature of power inside the ward, and as this chapter goes on to show, this ability does not always result in negative outcomes for patients.

What is surveillance?

Lyon (2017: 824) suggests that an "unprecedented surveillance culture is emerging", where people participate to regulate not only the surveillance of others but also their own surveillance. Therefore, it is not just sufficient to say "where surveillance is happening. We need some explanations of why surveillance is proliferating today, what is behind it, and who is affected" (Lyon, 2007: 2). The word surveillance, according to Lyon, comes from the French word "surveiller", meaning to "watch over". He defines surveillance as the "focused, systematic and routine attention to personal details for the purpose of influence, management, protection or direction" (Lyon, 2007: 14). This, he claims, includes everything from face-to-face encounters to surveillance using a range of information technologies. Lyon (2007) also suggests that the ambiguity of surveillance is manifest in its promotion of care and safety of those being watched as well as in the controlling of people whose behaviour may be under suspicion. As already stated, the observation or surveillance of patients inside mental health wards is not a new activity. Face-to-face surveillance of people is also a well-established practice within the caring field. Direct contact with patients and clients is fundamental to certain professions such as social work and nursing. Social work, for example, is based on individual casework, family work, group work and community work (Thompson, 2005). These interventions are reliant on face-to-face interactions and any challenges that these interactions bring with them. Similarly, medical examinations are also based on face-to-face encounters between a doctor and their patient. This contact is not just about a dialogue with the patient about symptoms; a face-to-face encounter allows the doctor to pick up non-verbal signs of distress, discomfort or when the patient is trying to conceal symptoms. Controlling people's behaviour through surveillance activities, therefore, can also be about enabling people to live fulfilled lives. For example, social work intervention may enable families to stay together and medical interventions allow people to live in their communities despite having a severe mental health condition. This caring aspect of surveillance is informed by a different set of ethics and principles where the motivation for intervention is based on the empowerment of people whether that empowerment is from abuse, distress or frightening thoughts and beliefs.

Haggerty and Ericson (2007: 4) suggest that surveillance "is a feature of modernity" and that it is "integral to the development of disciplinary power, modern subjectivities, and technologies of governance". They claim that whilst technological developments and computerised data systems have increased our awareness of surveillance, surveillance itself does not lead to the effective management of the state and that it needs to cohere with other agendas, for example, "rational governance, risk management, scientific progress, and military conquest" (2007: 4). Similarly, the mental health ward is also impacted by a range of agendas that often work together. For example, the locking down of mental health wards not only works as an effective security measure in that it stops unscrupulous members of the public who want to take advantage of vulnerable patients inside it. It also works as an effective safety tool in preventing patients from absconding from the ward. Wilkie et al. (2014) claim that absconsion from a hospital is not only a safety concern but also a health concern, resulting in the potential setback of a patient's treatment and recovery. Therefore, the one act of locking the ward results in maintaining security by keeping people out, as a safety tool by keeping patients in and as a health tool because it assists recovery. Therefore, each new way of surveilling the ward, whether that is through CCTV cameras, body-worn cameras or covert filming as sanctioned by the Care Quality Commission (2014) (England and Wales), is not limited to the task that they were authorised. They also cohere to other agendas that currently remain unknown because their full uses have yet to be discovered. What also remains unknown is how these tools also impact the more "pastoral and productive" forms of surveillance described by Moore (2011: 257).

Sovereign power and panoptic power

Theoretical perspectives related to CCTV have centred on what the media have labelled as the "Big Brother" society, where Big Brother (based on Orwell's "*Ninety Eighty-Four*" novel), an all-seeing leader, known only as Big Brother (a character who may not even exist), watches and scrutinises the private and public lives of the people of Oceania, through ubiquitous television or "telescreens". Academics and researchers have also been drawn to Foucault's interpretation of Jeremy Bentham's architectural design of a prison, named by Bentham as the Panopticon. Within the Panopticon, uncertainty is created among prisoners who are unaware as to whether they are being watched or not, which serves "to induce in the inmate a state of conscious and permanent visibility that assures the automatic functioning of power" (Foucault, 1979: 201). Foucault claimed that it did not matter whether the inmate was being watched or not. What mattered was whether the inmate believed that they were being watched and as a result conformed their behaviour as if they were being watched. This exercise of power on the individual or groups of patients is done to develop their ability to control their behaviour to the norms of society.

Prior to community care policies in the early 1990s, the care of people with mental health needs was predominantly inside asylums. Foucault (1971) believed that it is the confinement of madness that has led to the medical surveillance of such people. However, he did not believe that the emergence of the mental health institution was due to careful design and organisation. Foucault suggested that this emergence was based on maritime and military models where the prime function was not to seek a cure for madness. It was instead to bring the patient back to their senses so that they could continue to be a productive citizen in society. Foucault (1979) suggested that the influence of the maritime hospital was concerned with quarantine, resulting in patients inside it not being able to discharge themselves from it in the same way as they can do so in a general hospital. The military influence was the use of continuous surveillance inside these institutions to ensure that patients were not faking their illness. It was the exposure of the patient body in this way that, as Foucault suggests, led to the discovery of the body as an "object and target of power" (Foucault, 1979: 136). Asylums and post-institutional mental health hospitals still have these aspects of the maritime and military features, where patients are quarantined inside hospitals through legal detention under mental health legislation, and when inside, by being placed under continuous observation. For Foucault, it was the techniques used by the military in manipulating bodies that resulted in the rise of hierarchical, continuous and functional surveillance. He also believed that it was through the application of this surveillance that "disciplinary power became an 'integrated' system" (Foucault, 1979: 176). The mental health hospital, together with other institutions such as schools, factories and prisons, became a spatial apparatus in which disciplinary processes are operated.

Military influences were not restricted to disciplinary power. Asylums and post-institutional mental health hospitals also endorse the use of sovereign power. Foucault (1979) claimed that sovereign power is based on hierarchical power that is asserted through the Crown or other agents and that when sovereign power operates, the person on whom it is acted on knows not only who is acting upon them but also why. Asylums were well known for a range of practices, such as the heavy use of seclusion, forced medication, use of ECT (or electroconvulsive therapy where the patient has small electrical currents passed through their brain to induce a seizure), physical restraints and the carrying out of lobotomies (where part of the brain is removed or operated on so that certain behaviours or thought patterns can be eradicated). Some of these practices, for example, lobotomies (now known as neurosurgery), are hardly practised inside modern mental health hospitals, and when they are used, strict procedures are applied. These practices share similar characteristics in that they are about physical intervention on the patient body in which the patient has very little or no influence in what is done to them. This form of hierarchical power, according to Foucault (1979), required continuous action on the patient body, whereas disciplinary power could be exhibited through spatial and temporal dimensions. For example, space can be divided to

> establish presences and absences, to know where and how to locate individuals, to set up useful communication, to interrupt others, to be able at each moment supervise the conduct of each individual, to assess it, to judge it, to calculate its qualities or merits.
>
> (Foucault, 1979: 143)

The mental health hospital or asylum was perceived as the perfect apparatus in the constant surveillance of the patient because the hospital remains the perfect space in which to continuously observe patients and shape their behaviour.

For Foucault (2008), the most effective form of disciplinary power was panoptic power. He believed that a mental health hospital is a panoptic machine because its primary function is to cure madness or to bring it under control. He identified four panoptic features which can be applied to asylums and modern mental health hospitals. These include permanent visibility, central supervision, isolation and punishment. For him, the panoptic aspect of the asylum and modern mental health hospital is created by breaking off contact not only with the outside world but also with the patient's family. Inside the asylum, the patient must always be visible:

> The madman [*sic*] must not only be someone who is watched; the fact of knowing that one is always being watched, better still the fact of knowing that one can always be watched, that one is always under the potential power of a permanent gaze, has therapeutic value itself.
>
> (Foucault, 2008: 102)

Foucault believed that it is the point at which the patient realises that they are looked at as mad that they will no longer display their madness. This does not mean that the patient who, for example, is delusional and who believes that they are God will no longer believe this. Cure in the context of the mental health ward is not just about challenging a patient's perception and belief. It is also about not openly vocalising that they are God (whether they believe this or not), and it certainly is not about conducting their behaviour as if they were God. To be satisfied that the patient understands this, Foucault (2008: 102) believed that they "must be in a position of someone who can always be seen". Therefore, the hospital as a panoptic curing machine is not only satisfied with scrutinising a patient's thoughts and feelings, but their behaviour must also come under scrutiny.

According to Foucault, the distillation of these disciplinary techniques, that is, permanent visibility, central supervision, isolation and punishment, is to be found in Bentham's design of the Panopticon or Inspection-House. Božovič (1995) describes through Bentham's letters how Bentham intended to build a prison, based on his brother's original plans for an Inspection-House or Elaboratory in London. Bentham believed that his Inspection-House was not only applicable to prison (or correction houses), but its design could also be applied to "workhouses, or manufactories, or mad-houses, or hospitals, or schools" (Božovič, 1995: 34). Bentham describes the design of the Inspection-House as circular with cells surrounding its circumference, where each prisoner is unable to communicate with another. At the centre of this circumference is the inspector's lodge from which the supervisor maintains a watchful gaze over the inmates. The essence of Bentham's Inspection-House is that the supervisor can see the prisoner, without the prisoner being able to see the supervisor. This creates uncertainty among prisoners about who is watching them, when they are watched and what is watched, making supervision a more intense experience. It is not knowing whether someone is watching or not, which creates constant and absolute visibility of bodies.

Foucault (1979) believed that this generates a particular psychological belief in the mind of those being watched, where they are deceived into thinking that they are under constant surveillance. Although Bentham's ideal prison or mental hospital never materialised, Foucault himself wrote, "the panopticon must not be understood as a dream building: it is the diagram of a mechanism of power reduced to its ideal form" (1979: 205).

Foucault did not provide a detailed account of how panoptic power operated inside mental health hospitals, especially in the context of day-to-day practices and techniques used inside it. Goffman's (1961) description of life inside asylums to date remains one of the few comprehensive studies on the techniques and practices used inside asylums to control patient behaviour. These techniques and practices incorporate a range of processes that the patient is required to feel as well as experience. They, therefore, are not just about mundanely engaging in practices and adhering to ward rules, they are also about processes by which patients understand their subordinate position within the ward. For example, Goffman (1961: 45) claimed that patients were placed in "submissive or suppliant role 'unnatural' for an adult", where acts such as requesting to smoke a cigarette or going to the shop placed the patient in a submissive role with staff which would be open to the request being "denied, questioned at length, not noticed". He describes how admission procedures involved the taking of a person's life history, physical body searches of patients, the listing of a person's possessions and so on. These procedures, according to Goffman, ignored the patient's previous status in life before becoming a patient, and rather than individual people who required guidance and inspection, Goffman believed that patients were instead treated as "whole blocks" (1961: 18). Smaller staff teams effectively managed large groups of patients where "everyone does what he [*sic*] has been clearly told is required of him [*sic*], under conditions where one person's infraction is likely to stand out in relief against the visible, constantly examined compliance of the others" (Goffman, 1961: 18). Isolation of patients was achieved by restricted communication among patients, and between staff and patients.

The role of staff was to maintain a watchful eye over large groups of patients, where this involvement did not require any emotional engagement with them. In addition, this watchful gaze was not an empathic gaze, and the disindividualisation of patients in this way was to show them that they were not unique, because they believed that they were God, related to royalty, were royalty or have any other delusional or distorted ideas. For their part, patients, even where they did not like being treated this way, accepted ward rules because being "normal" means that they are no longer perceived as "abnormal", and more importantly, they can no longer be marginalised as such. It is by showing that they can conform to asylum rules that they can prove to others that they have the ability to control their behaviour. This is known as having "insight" into their mental health condition. Gaining insight means that they know that their behaviour is abnormal or that their thought process is disordered. It is this insight that suggests that they are "cured", or their behaviour corrected enough so as not to need the hospital any longer. It is through this that Foucault (1979: 203) claimed the patient becomes "the principle of his [*sic*] own subjection". This is because the patient has been able to internalise the rules of the wider society, where normal behaviour does not include people openly claiming that they are God or behaving as if they were God. It is the ability of the patient to regulate their behaviour, even when their behaviour is not causing any harm to other people or themselves, that they can demonstrate to others they can exercise power over themselves. Haggerty and Ericson (2000: 607) suggest that this "disciplinary aspect of panoptic observation involves a productive soul training which encourages inmates to reflect upon the minutia of their own behaviour in subtle and ongoing efforts to transform their selves". This psyche or soul training results in the internalisation of "normal" behaviours and ultimately in self-discipline where there is no need for walls (Bogard, 2006).

Although the panoptic aspect of visibility and disciplinary power is recognisable through standardised living activities and nurse observation, these were not the only way in which asylums controlled patient behaviours. The behavioural model adopted inside asylums also relied on punishment or the threat of punishment, for example, through the practices of seclusion, forcible medication and physical restraint. These practices, which are reminiscent of sovereign power, are still practised inside modern mental health hospitals. While panoptic power is more interested in patient behaviour and understanding the characteristics of their behaviour, sovereign power is about controlling patient behaviour when they are perceived as being unable to do so for themselves. Inside mental health wards, patients are not always able to understand the panoptic aspect of disciplinary power. This is because their mental health condition can impact their capacity to understand the subtleties of panoptic power. Controlling the patient's behaviour therefore cannot be entirely reliant on the use of panoptic power in shaping their behaviour. The use of seclusion practice, forced medication and physical restraint are tactics that continue to be used inside modern mental hospitals. These practices are not used to punish the patient, although patients who experience seclusion, forced medication and physical restraint believe that these forces on the body are akin to punishment (Keski-Valkama et al., 2010). They are used as part of a therapeutic intervention to bring the patient's behaviour under control. How sovereign power and panoptic power are played out in the context of the modern mental health ward is dependent upon pastoral power and the understanding of interventions that are likely to bring about the best outcomes for patients.

Pastoral power

Foucault (2009) places the consultant psychiatrist at the centre of the distillation of power inside the mental health ward. According to him, pastoral power has three significant identifying features. First, he attributes pastoral power to the body of the psychiatrist who, he claims, creates a dissymmetry in the asymmetrical surveillance operating inside the ward, where the psychiatrist is not concerned with the acquisition of territory (that is the ward) and instead has, as her or his focal point, the acquisition or well-being of the flock (the patients). Second, Foucault claims that pastoral power is "fundamentally a beneficent power", where it is the responsibility of the consultant psychiatrist to ensure that patients are safe and well cared for, and therefore "pastoral power is a power of care" (Foucault, 2009: 126). Thirdly, how well patients are cared for inside the ward is down to the individualising power of the psychiatrist and her or his ability to be a good doctor, who works for the best outcomes for their patients. Sovereign power relies on the control of the patient body through the ability of staff and the psychiatrist to impose their will over the patient, for example, by forcing them to be placed into seclusion or deciding that they need to be sedated through forced medication. Pastoral power is reliant on relational power. It is the ability inside the ward, for example, to persuade the patient to take their medication as opposed to forcing it upon them or, it is the ability to engage the patient in monitoring their behaviour, feelings and thoughts and in managing these in ways that allow them to lead a normal life away from the hospital (Barker, 1997). In this way, pastoral power in the context of the ward is also temporary where the relationship between the patient and staff has relevancy only in the context of the patient's time inside the ward.

Pastoral power operates for the well-being of others and how well the consultant psychiatrist and ward staff work for the benefit of each patient. Although Foucault has primarily drawn on the figure of the consultant psychiatrist in his distillation of pastoral power, nursing literature has also highlighted the importance of building relationships with patients (through, for example, person-centred care) as an essential part of recovery, rather than the containment of patients inside the ward (Barker, 2001; Bowers et al., 2015; Edal et al., 2019). This view is based on the recognition that patients want staff to acknowledge them as people has evolved since Peplau (1952) claimed that interpersonal relationships are central to mental health nursing. Edal et al. (2019) identify six significant features of interpersonal relationships between staff and their patients. Some of these include a values base that recognises the patient as a person and not as a diagnosis, expectations based on consistency which relies on getting to know one or a few staff very well and the ability to establish relationships with staff who are knowledgeable. Patient experiences inside mental health wards often differ. This is because each hospital and each ward has a specific culture within it which is influenced not only by the consultant psychiatrist and those staff who work inside it but also by the organisational culture. For example, some wards choose not to use seclusion as a means of controlling patient behaviour, where these wards do not have any designated seclusion room, de-escalation room or access to seclusion facilities in other wards. Staff on these wards manage patient behaviour by talking to patients and calming them down or allowing them to have time out inside their bedroom, or other ward spaces and also sometimes through medication. Inside modern mental health wards, it is not only the consultant psychiatrist who provides leadership, the ward manager and the nurse in charge also influences how patient care should be administered, especially on a day-to-day basis. Unlike asylums which perceive patients as blocks of people, most modern mental health wards operate by recognising that each patient is an individual with a different worldview and that any intervention with patients has to be at a personal level to affect change. It is this aspect of relational or pastoral power that separates the modern mental hospital from the asylum.

According to Foucault pastoral power is an extension of disciplinary power, which provides an alternative inside the ward to sovereign power (Dreyfus and Rabinow, 1983). This is because pastoral power is productive power. Inside the ward, pastoral power is not static; it circulates in ways that influence patient behaviour, sometimes through kindness, sometimes through punishment and sometimes through the process of ignoring the patient. In this manner, Foucault (2008) suggests that pastoral power has links with Judeo-Christian tradition, where the pastor aims to modify the spirit of the guided person through confessions. The role of the consultant psychiatrist is to enable the patient to gain insight into their mental health condition by showing the patient the errors of their way and guide the patient back to wellness. In this way, the patient begins to produce a truth about themselves, where even if they do believe that they have blue hair and blue blood and are a direct descendant of the Queen, they know that they should not vocalise this or behave in ways that suggest they are royalty. While panoptic power relies on the uncertainty of knowing or not knowing when one is being looked at, pastoral power relies on the therapeutic relationship between the patient and their psychiatrist (and staff) in shaping behaviour, and similar to panoptic power, it is reliant on the invisibility of power. However, both target the patient body for the same purpose.

Sovereign power, panoptic power and pastoral power

In his lectures at the Collège de France, Foucault (2009) introduced the concept of governmentality where he has located the functions of pastoral power to political institutions. The function of governmentality is, according to Foucault (2009), based on how we govern ourselves and other people. The pastoral aspect of governmentality is not based on hierarchical control of power and is instead based on the concerns of the whole population as well as each individual within it. Foucault (2009: xix) believed that governmentality was reliant on managing conduct or "conducting conduct":

> Conduct is the activity of conducting (*conduire*), of conduction (*la conduction*) if you like, but it is equally the way in which one conducts oneself (*se conduit*), lets oneself be conducted (*se laisse conduire*), and finally, in which one behaves (*se comporter*) under the influence of a conduct as the action of conducting or of conduction (*conduction*).

According to him, power can only be exercised on those people who believe that they are a "free subject". In order to normalise behaviour, populations and people have to be disciplined in a certain way. The framework for analysis adopted in this research examines the interplay between sovereign power, panoptic power and pastoral power in conducting and discipling the patient's behaviour. This analysis is not about who has the power to control the behaviour and actions of the patient inside the ward. It is about the relations of power adopted inside the mental health ward which include a range of techniques and technologies of power in influencing and shaping patient behaviour. Whereas asylum care was about governing patients because of the permanency of such hospital care, modern mental health hospitals are about governing the self. Success for modern mental health hospitals lies in their ability to persuade the patient to govern themselves. The modern mental hospital is different because it is not concerned with controlling the patient; it sees itself as a temporary measure in the recovery of the patient.

Disciplining of patient behaviours according to the norms of society are therefore reliant on the careful functioning of sovereign power, panoptic power and pastoral power inside the ward. The use of techniques (such as nurse monitoring) and other practices are impacted when new technology is added because it can potentially change the balance of power inside the ward. This is because any new technology can cohere to agendas that may or may not benefit the patient. For example, cameras have the potential to impact therapeutic relationships inside the ward because they have the potential to open up new ways of observing patient behaviours that previously relied on face-to-face encounters. The ability to observe patients in an unobtrusive way using the cameras makes the behaviour being observed more authentic and objective because the patient does not always know whether they are seen or what is seen. This objectivity influences the analysis of the mental health condition because it allows staff to focus on diagnostic characteristics for the patient's behaviour. This not only has the potential to define the patient in the context of their diagnosis, where they are no longer seen as a person. It can also lead to a misinterpretation of what is happening as the behaviour is viewed out of context. In addition, as the cameras influence the panoptic nature of watching inside the ward, they also impact other aspects. For instance, the loss of in-person contact with patients can also influence staff and how they perceive the job. In this way, for some staff, each day becomes a matter of surviving the shift, as opposed to finding job fulfilment through interaction with patients and colleagues in a meaningful way. This creates a gap between the nurse as a "custodian" and the nurse as a "therapeutic" agent of control (Marshall and Adam, 2018).

The shift in power through the addition of cameras inside the ward can also impact how psychiatry is practised inside it, including the leadership aspirations of the consultant psychiatrist. While some consultant psychiatrists might prefer psychotherapeutic or psychoanalytic approaches to understand patient behaviour, the organisational or institutional goals related to patient care may not necessarily support this. As mental health hospitals become sensitive to how others perceive them, the availability of the cameras inside the ward offers opportunities to exonerate themselves from negative public opinion. Mental health research and literature draw heavily on the violent nature of the patient, where hospitals are perceived as unsafe places to be inside (see, for example, Whittington and Ritcher, 2006; Bowers et al., 2011; Stevenson et al., 2015). Whether this is true for all mental health wards in all hospitals becomes irrelevant. What becomes the practice is that an incident inside one hospital will lead to a "knee-jerk" response (as described by one manager in Chapter 3) where all hospitals have to increase surveillance of patients or staff, or of visitors to the ward. The ward space therefore also becomes a place where organisational and managerial anxieties are also played out, where the watching of the patient becomes about continuously assessing their risky behaviour. These aspects influence how patients are perceived and where managerial influences undermine pastoral care; they also change the nature of how patient behaviour is interpreted. It is therefore important to understand how power plays out inside the ward environment and how the addition of practices and tools (such as CCTV, body-worn cameras or sanctioning of covert filming as evidence) changes the nature of the ward.

This research has adopted Foucault's framework of sovereign power, panoptic power and pastoral power in the governance of patients inside the ward to highlight how various practices and relationships inside the ward are influenced by the presence of CCTV cameras. To understand how the cameras can change the nature of mental health care inside the ward, the empirical data chapters also draw on a range of other theoretical perspectives. These theoretical perspectives show how sovereign power, panoptic power and pastoral power become embedded inside the ward. For example, the Social Construction of Technology or the SCOT approach (Pinch and Bijker , 2012) politicises the implementation of the cameras and their ability to produce a range of outcomes dependent on their social circumstances. Ellul's (1964) theoretical analysis of "*technique*" highlights how unreflective behaviour can become rationalised into everyday practices inside the ward. Levinas's (2006) analysis of the loss of face as staff become invisible inside the ward and the impact of the imagined (or hidden) presence of cameras in shaping behaviour, as highlighted by Latané (1981), are also influential in how patient conduct is shaped. Also, the figure of the consultant psychiatrist has not been examined in the context of her or his influence in shaping the patient's behaviour. Therefore, the empirical data draws on these additional theoretical concepts to examine how the cameras influence and shape patient behaviours.

Post-Panopticon

Surveillant assemblage

Deleuze and Guattari suggest that the range of techniques, technologies and procedures that are adopted inside mental health wards, despite at times seeming divergent, form a "fragmentary whole" (cited in Nail, 2017: 23). This fragmentary whole, according to them, does not constitute a whole picture as in pieces of a jigsaw puzzle but is more like a dry-stone wall where everything is held together along divergent lines forming its own assemblage. Each new addition such as CCTV or body-worn cameras produces a new assemblage or a new line of surveillance. Therefore, the cameras may have been introduced inside the ward to manage security, for example, to question anyone inside the ward who should not be there. However, as other issues arise inside the ward, such as a dispute between a patient and staff, the availability of CCTV footage which can also be used to resolve these issues leads to the expanded uses of cameras. It is in this way that the cameras begin to cohere with other agendas inside the ward. The expansion of camera use is not just limited to resolving disputes that happen inside the ward, for example, staff might also use them to do unobtrusive watching of patient behaviour to gain a better understanding of their mental health condition, or managers might use them to watch staff and make sure that they are doing the job properly. Therefore, camera use is not restricted to resolving or understanding a crisis; they can also easily slip into everyday practices and concerns inside the ward. Previous research into the use of CCTV cameras has also shown how the cameras are used for more than their intended purpose. Warr et al. (2005), for example, found that bedroom cameras intended for carrying out unobtrusive night-time observations of patients while they were sleeping were also used by staff for other purposes. For instance, staff in their study also used the cameras to see if a patient's behaviour in their bedroom differed from their presentation in the communal areas of the ward. Although this use of the cameras in the bedroom was not sanctioned, staff justified their use for this purpose because they claimed that the cameras allowed them to "get a snapshot picture" of the patient's presentation, which at times was different from how they behaved in the communal areas of the ward (Warr et al., 2005: 25). Warr et al. demonstrate how easy it is to change the function and use of cameras as they adhere to other agendas inside the ward.

Similarly, in an internal review of the cameras for their NHS Mental Health Trust, Chambers and Gillard (2005) describe how the use of cameras impacted staff–patient relationships. According to them, some nursing staff were reluctant to use therapeutic touch with patients in case their actions were deemed to be inappropriate by managers when they reviewed any CCTV footage. However, while some staff were reticent about using touch, other staff claimed that they felt more confident about using physical intervention with patients such as restraining them because these staff believed that any video footage would show that they had intervened appropriately. These examples suggest that not only do the cameras change behaviour in unintended ways, but they can also change the therapeutic environment inside the ward. Chambers and Gillard's review suggests that techniques and practices based on sovereign power have the potential to increase inside the ward because staff have the confidence in using full-body restraint of the patient, where the intervention becomes about the mechanics of doing restraint as opposed to why restraint was necessary or how it could have been avoided. These examples suggest that while the cameras are part of a network of practices in the ward that is about keeping patients safe, their uses are not fixed. Therefore, the use of bedroom cameras by staff to examine patient behaviour out of sanctioned times in their bedroom, as shown in Warr et al.'s (2005) study, was not perceived by them as inappropriate. DeLanda (2006) suggests that this is because there is no pre-determined logic to how assemblages connect and that the only thing that unites them is their ability to co-function with other agendas. Chapters 3 and 4 explore a range of practices and uses of cameras that are linked to risk, violence, medical surveillance, politics and efficacy in relation to doing the job, which determines how the cameras are used inside the ward.

Haggerty and Ericson (2000) have drawn on Deleuze and Guattari's description of assemblages to describe how they increase surveillance. For instance, they suggest that the appeal of the surveillant assemblage is that it is neither hierarchical nor asymmetrical. They draw on Deleuze and Guattari's description of the rhizome plant to claim that the rhizome plant can reproduce through the process of interconnected root systems which results in horizontal surveillance. More importantly, it is this ability of the surveillant assemblage to expand surveillance to those people who previously were not the focus of attention, which also results in the levelling effect of surveillance. Inside the ward, cameras are not only used to judge the behaviour of patients, they are also used to judge the behaviour of staff. Mann et al. (2003: 332) coined the term sousveillance or inverse surveillance to "challenge and problematize" surveillance through the use of surveillance technologies in observing those people in authority. They suggest that the use of surveillance technologies in this way offers people, who are not in a position of authority, the opportunity to resist surveillance from such authorities. For example, it can show that a patient behaved appropriately in a given situation, which before the availability of visual footage would have relied on verbal accounts offered by staff and patients, where often patients felt that their account was considered as less credible by those in authority (Staniszewska et al., 2019).

CCTV footage can also be used by the patient's family and groups that are interested in exposing abuse inside mental health wards and hospitals. Two documentaries, Whorlton Hall (BBC 1, 2019) and Winterbourne View (BBC 1, 2011), both private mental health hospitals in which patient abuse was revealed by undercover exposure, which were televised in a documentary television programme titled "Panorama", are examples of how covert camera use can expose poor practices by staff. These practices may not have become known, or even where they were known by staff and managers at the hospitals been exposed to the wider world without covert filming. Therefore, the appeal of the cameras to patients who are the initial target of CCTV surveillance is that they have an added advantage when proving to others that they were the victims of violence or aggressive acts done to them by staff and occasionally other patients. These uses of the cameras increase their appeal to patients, families or carers of the patient, managers and staff inside the ward because their uses are not limited to the concerns of one group.

Deleuze and Guattri (1980) also suggest that assemblages abstract the human body from its territorial setting by separating them into discrete flows. They claim that assemblages are created by multiple heterogeneous objects. These objects work together to form a functional entity and that if one were to investigate what was beneath a particular assemblage or heterogeneous object, one would find "discrete flows of essentially limitless range of other phenomena such as people, signs, chemicals, knowledge and institutions" (Haggerty and Ericson, 2000: 606–608). For the subjects of surveillance, this abstraction of the human body into discrete flows has several implications because it reduces patient behaviours into discrete parts, such as their triggers to violence, their propensity for violence, which parts of the communal areas of the ward they become violent in, what they do when they believe they are being watched, how they behave when they are not and so on. This reduction of the patient as body movements changes the nature of care inside the ward because the patient is no longer seen as a whole person. The reduction of their body movements into these different parts are justified on the basis that it helps in the nursing of patients and the more that is known about each person's behaviour the better it is because staff can then predict when the patient is likely to become hostile and aggressive and intervene before the situation gets out of hand (see Chapter 4). This abstraction of the patient body into discrete flows, which allow staff to manage and understand each patient behaviour in their care, is not only limited to this. The ability to manage patient hostility inside mental health hospitals is also critical to wider political agendas and the hospital's reputation. These aspects are also critical to the survival of the hospital.

Big Brother and Little Sisters

In the post-Panopticon era, Romein and Schuilenburg suggest that rather than "Big Brother" surveillance, what has emerged is "Little Sisters".

According to them, these forms of surveillance are driven by "numerous dispersed surveillant assemblages that are playing an important role in the control of our behaviour" (2008: 344). They also suggest that modern surveillance methods such as the use of CCTV cameras and body-worn cameras are concerned with dividing, categorising and excluding. However, how they divide, categorise and exclude happen in very subtle ways. Bauman suggests that modern surveillance practices require being united in the act of watching or being seduced into it (Bauman cited in Boyne, 2000). Mathiesen (1997), for example, has coined the term synopticon to introduce the notion of the viewer society where the many watch the few. Within synoptic surveillance, watching is not limited to the influence created by Big Brother, who may or may not exist. Watching instead becomes the prerogative of the many. This is not based on a deficit model, where a medical practitioner (such as a general practitioner or psychiatrist) confirms that there is something wrong with a person's mind. It is based on how the public seeks fulfilment through aspects related to mental health, mental well-being, happiness and positive emotional health. It is also influenced by an understanding of how certain aspects like stress can induce mental health problems. In this way, Boyne (2000: 299) argues that contemporary British society is not only about the few watching the many but is also "marked by the phenomenon of very large numbers watching the activities of the very few". For him, repeated exposure to media society connect to our own "self-identification and self-understanding" of a range of concerns, including mental health issues. For example, through exposure to television documentaries about mental health conditions, mental health depictions and storylines linked to certain characters within television soap operas, and by the reporting of mental health issues and mental health campaigns in the news, press and magazines. These aspects impact how we develop our understanding of what it means to be normal. This exposure also influences how as a society we understand mental health issues and how we engage in our self-surveillance practices, by determining what is perceived as normal behaviour and what might be perceived as abnormal behaviour.

Similarly, Deleuze (1992) also suggests that Foucault's panoptic society is increasingly being replaced by societies of control. Deleuze suggests that societies of control operate with technological machines such as CCTV. CCTV cameras are not only to be found inside mental health wards, they are also found within other sectors, including workplaces, schools, nurseries and so on (see the previous chapter). Their uses are therefore extensive. However, unlike Foucault's (1979) panopticism based on the uncertainty of watching, Deleuze suggests that in societies of control, people know that they are being watched and are encouraged not to worry about this as surveillance becomes more normalised. Also, Foucault (1979) believed that people pass from one disciplinary environment to another, for example, the family, the school, the workplace, sometimes the hospital and/or the prison where each has its laws and rules. Deleuze (1992) suggests that in the post-Panopticon era, the lines that distinguish the hospital from the community are less stable. The actions, behaviours and bodies of people with mental health conditions are therefore not only surveilled within the walls of the hospital, but they are also surveilled through formal policy interventions via the numerous mental health and other services designed to keep a watchful eye on them, including by patients themselves as targets of their own surveillance.

Government-based campaigns and policies, such as "Time to Change", informed by mental health charities and supported by the Department of Health and Social Care (2018), recognise this and enable patients to participate in their surveillance by encouraging them to monitor their progress and to seek help when they experience signs of relapse. These government and charity-led campaigns have resulted in the rise of a vast range of self-help and therapeutic models and interventions, for example, Wellness Recovery Action Planning (WRAP). These models have in common a self-help element, life-long learning and openness about one's mental health status. Recovery is not linked to curing and is based on the individualised meaning that is not necessarily about being symptomless, but about learning to control the negative symptoms of their mental health condition (Ryan et al., 2012). Glover sums up the ethos behind recovery:

> Our responsibility is not to assess, manage, monitor, teach and rehabilitate, but to create environments where a person can recognise their mastery, and continue to learn and thrive beyond the limitations invited by the experience of mental illness or distress.
>
> (2012: 15)

The important aspect of Deleuze's (1992) societies of control is that mental health concerns are no longer confined to the hospital. The ability to master one's mental health creates a sense of freedom, although this freedom comes with challenges. For example, while this creates freedom from the mental health ward and its enclosed environment, it also creates the stress of constantly having to monitor one's behaviour, assessing whether this behaviour would be acceptable to others, curbing thoughts and beliefs to fit in. Societies of control, therefore, create the illusion that mental health concerns are normal and accepted. People are encouraged to talk more about their feelings and emotions and how these impact their mental well-being. This does not necessarily lead to acceptance of mental health concerns but more medicalisation of emotions as people begin to monitor all their behaviour more critically.

Post-institutional care is also reliant on the detection of symptoms and signs of madness through the early detection of mental health conditions. It is in the vested interest of medicine and psychiatry to support these political agendas which do not undermine their expertise. Mental health research founded on evidence-based medicine promoted since the early 1990s supports the claim that early medical intervention leads to better outcomes of recovery from mental illness. This has also influenced a rise in the number of professional and lay groups tasked with identifying people with potential mental health difficulties. These groups have extended well beyond Rose's (1989: 2) "new professional groups" of social workers and psychologists. These groups now include employers, university and college staff and school teachers whose role also involves seeking out and bringing to the attention of mental health professionals those people that they believe are showing signs of abnormal behaviour. For example, the UK government has placed a stipulation on mental health funding where it has prioritised the training of school teachers in recognising the early signs of mental health problems in pupils so that psychiatric intervention can happen early on (Gov.UK: Press Release, 27 June 2017). This agenda for surveilling young people for signs of mental illness also cohere with other agendas such as the identification of future potential political terrorists. These developments in mental health also share several similarities to other behaviours seen as deviant, including crime. Simon (2007: 5), for example, makes a distinction between "governing through crime", from "governing crime" where he claims that it is not only criminal justice organisations that are dedicated to dealing with the threat of crime in society, other institutions such as "families, schools and businesses, are also mobilised to act when crime threatens". This strategy, also adopted in mental health care, has not only widened its influence in engaging a range of people in the surveillance of madness, but it has also successfully cohered with other agendas. The widening of mental health surveillance in this way also produces greater inequalities because for young people, it has the potential for early medicalisation of their behaviour resulting in possibly life-long surveillance, through their early labelling as having a mental disorder.

Resistance

The fragmentation of surveillance and societal attitudes to being under surveillance suggests that resistance to surveillance is not an issue because we know we are being watched and we are not concerned about it. However, resisting camera surveillance inside the ward is not straightforward, and there are three key elements of camera surveillance that impact how patients might resist such surveillance. The first is linked to their mental health condition. For example, it cannot be assumed that patients who experience fluctuating cognitive distortions as a result of their mental health condition have the awareness and ability to understand the panoptic aspects of the cameras. Yar, for example, claims that if subjects of surveillance are not consciously aware of their visibility, then the relationship between "visibility and discipline collapses" (Yar, 2003: 260–261). Second, the cameras are not limited to mental health ward use. CCTV cameras are to be found everywhere; therefore, it is likely that they would find their way inside mental health wards, especially as a primary function of the ward is the observation of patients. Linked to this point is the third factor, which is that patients inside the mental health ward know that they are in the ward to be observed. In all three research sites, patients were given a patient information leaflet on admission which explained that they would be observed inside the ward. Therefore, most patients knew that the staff were there to observe them. Connected to this, several patients also believed that the cameras would be used to observe them. All these aspects influenced how patients resisted camera surveillance (discussed more fully in Chapter 5).

Resistance to camera surveillance, therefore, was not always based on collective action or through the use of formalised systems such as complaints procedures. They were based on what Johansson and Vinthagen (2014: 5) describe as individualised and collective actions that "are not organised, formal or necessarily public or intentionally political". Resistance to surveillance was also not influenced by the panoptic hierarchical nature of CCTV surveillance. This is because some patients welcomed the fact the ward had cameras so that when they were accused of wrongdoing, CCTV evidence would exonerate them. Camera resistance inside the mental health ward was primarily influenced by having relief from constant observation and surveillance of their behaviour as patients.

Marx (2009) has argued that new forms of surveillance have emerged as a result of Deleuzian societies of control, where power is both absent and dispersive. He has identified 11 forms of surveillance neutralisation (some of these are discussed in more detail in Chapter 5), which include: discovery moves, avoidance moves, piggybacking moves, switching moves, distorting moves, blocking moves, masking moves, breaking moves, refusal moves, cooperative moves and counter-surveillance moves. While these forms of surveillance neutralisation were linked to computerised work environments, some of these counter-surveillance moves have also been used by patients inside mental health hospitals. For example, detained patients inside mental health hospitals have used piggybacking moves by pretending to be a visitor or a staff member and following legitimate staff members or visitors out of the ward and very occasionally, successfully out of the hospital. Or cooperative moves which require cooperation with other patients such as one patient starting a fire in the ward to create a diversion so that other patients can attempt to abscond from it. Often these actions by patients are not perceived as resistance to surveillance but as disruptive behaviour which is sometimes linked to a patient's mental health condition and often to justify their detention inside the ward. Therefore, mental health literature has tended to ignore or undermine patient's attempts to escape from the ward or to disrupt surveillance in other ways as forms of resistance. This lack of documentation of ways in which patients resist surveillance inside the mental health ward has also meant that any "casual, unexpected, ironic, playful, and feeble" attempts at resistance have also remained undocumented (Ganesh, 2016: 168). Although it is not yet fully known how patients resist CCTV surveillance inside the ward, Marx claims that human beings "are wonderfully inventive at finding ways to beat control systems and to avoid observation" (2003: 372).

Conclusion

The analysis of CCTV cameras as a surveillance tool is subject to a range of theoretical perspectives. By drawing on a range of Panoptic and post-Panoptic theoretical perspectives, the chapter has laid out the basis on which camera implementation, camera use, cameras impact on the patient as a subject of surveillance and resistance to cameras will be explored in the subsequent three chapters. This chapter suggests that the ward is not defined by one type of power, for example, panoptic power and that any analysis of power inside the mental health ward has to consider the impact of sovereign power and pastoral power in the disciplining of a patient's behaviour.

Bibliography

Barker, P. (1997). *Assessment in Psychiatric Mental Health Nursing*, Cheltenham: Stanley Thornes Publishers.

Barker, P. (2001). "The tidal model: The lived-experience in person-centered mental health nursing care," *Nursing Philosophy*, 2(3): 213–223.

Bogard, W. (2006). "Surveillance assemblages and lines of flight," in D. Lyon (ed), *Theorising Surveillance: The Panopticon and Beyond*, Portland: Willan Publishing, pp.97–123.

Bowers, L., Alexander, J., Bilgin, H., Botha, M., Dack, C., James, K., Jarrett, M., Jeffery, D., Nijman, H., Owiti, J.A., Papadopoulos, C., Ross, J., Wright, S. and Stewart, D. (2014). "Safewards: The empirical basis of the model and a critical appraisal," *Journal of Psychiatric and Mental Health Nursing*, 21(4): 354–364.

Bowers, L., James, K., Quirk, A., Simpson, A., SUGAR, Stewart, D. and Hodsoll, J. (2015). "Reducing conflict and containment rates on acute psychiatric wards: The Safewards cluster randomised controlled trial," *International Journal of Nursing Studies*, 52(9): 1412–1422.

Boyne, R. (2000). "Post-panopticism," *Economy and Society*, 29(2): 285–307.

Božovič, M. (1995). *The Panoptic Writings: Jeremy Bentham*, London: Verso.

British Broadcasting Company (BBC 1). *Undercover Care: The Abuse Exposed, Winterbourne View*, Panorama, 31 May 2011.

British Broadcasting Company (BBC 1). *Undercover Hospital Abuse Scandal, Whorlton Hall*, Panorama, 22 May 2019.

Care Quality Commission (CQC). (2014). *Monitoring the Mental Health Act in 2013/14*, London: Care Quality Commission HMSO.

Chambers, M. and Gillard, S. (2005). *Review of CCTV on John Meyer Ward, 19 July 2005 Agenda Item 9, South West London and St George's NHS Mental Health Trust*, South West London and St George's NHS Mental Health Trust Board Meeting, 28 July 2005, London.

DeLanda, M. (2006). *A New Philosophy of Society: Assemblage Theory and Social Complexity, The Tower Building*, London: Continuum.

Deleuze, G. (1992). "Postscript on the societies of control," *October*, 59: 3–7.
Deluze, G. and Guattari, F. (1980). *A Thousand Plateaus*, translated by Brian Massumi, New York: University of Minnesota Press.
Department of Health and Social Care. (2018). *Time to Change*, Mind and Rethink Mental Illness. Available online: www.time-to-change.org.uk [accessed 10 October 2018].
Dreyfus, H.L. and Rabinow, P. (1983). *Michel Foucault: Beyond Structuralism and Hermeneutics. 2nd Edition. With an Afterword by an Interview with Michel Foucault*, Chicago: The University of Chicago Press.
Edal, K., Natvik, E., Veseth, M., Davidson, L., Skjolberg, A., Dorte, G. and Moltu, C. (2019). "Being recognised as a whole person: A qualitative study of inpatient experience in mental health," *Issues in Mental Health Nursing*, 40(2): 88–96.
Ellul, J. (1964). *The Technological Society*, New York: Vintage Books.
Foucault, M. (1971). *Madness and Civilization: A History of Insanity in the Age of Reason*, New York: Pantheon.
Foucault, M. (1979). *Discipline and Punish: The Birth of the Prison*, New York: Vintage.
Foucault, M. (2008). *Psychiatric Power: Lectures at the Collège de France 1973–1974*, edited by Jacques Lagrange and translated by Graham Burchell, Basingstoke: Palgrave.
Foucault, M. (2009). *Security, Territory, Population: Lectures at the Collège de France 1977–1978*, edited by Michel Senellart and translated by Graham Burchell, Basingstoke: Palgrave.
Ganesh, S. (2016). "Managing surveillance: Surveillant individualism in an era of relentless visibility," *International Journal of Communication*, 10: 164–177.
Gastaldo, D. and Holmes, D. (1999). "Foucault and nursing: A history of the present," *Nursing Inquiry*, 6(4): 231–240.
Gilburt, H., Rose, D. and Slade, M. (2008). "The importance of relationships in mental health care: A qualitative study of service users' experiences of psychiatric hospital admission in the UK," *BMC Health Service Research,* 8(92): 1–12. Available online: www.biomedcentral.com/1472-6963/8/92 [accessed 8 May 2019].
Glover, H. (2012). "Recovery, lifelong learning, empowerment and social inclusion: Is a new paradigm emerging?" in P. Ryan, S. Ramon and T. Greacen (eds), *Empowerment, Lifelong Learning and Recovery in Mental Health*, Basingstoke: Palgrave Macmillan, pp. 15–36.
Goffman, E. (1961). *Asylums: Essays on the Social Situation of Mental Patients and Other Inmates*, New York: Anchor Books.
Gov.UK: Press Release 27 June 2017 PM. *Mental Health Training for Teachers Will "Make a Real Difference to Children's Lives"*. Available online: www.gov.uk/government/news [accessed 23 January 2018].
Haggerty, K.D. and Ericson, R.V. (2000). "The surveillant assemblage," *British Journal of Sociology*, 51(4): 605–622.
Haggerty, K.D. and Ericson, R.V. (eds) (2007). *The New Politics Surveillance and Visibility*, Toronto, Buffalo, London: University of Toronto Press.
Holmes, D. (2001). "From iron gaze to nursing care: Mental health nursing in the era of the panopticism," *Journal of Psychiatric and Mental Health Nursing*, 8(1): 7–15.
Johansson, A. and Vinthagen, S. (2014). "Dimensions of everyday resistance: An analytical framework," *Critical Sociology*, 42(3): 417–435.
Kesey, K. (1973). *One Flew Over the Cuckoo's Nest*, London: Pan Books.

Keski-Valkama, A., Koivisto, A-M, Eronen, M. and Kaltiala-Heino, R. (2010). "Forensic and general psychiatric patients' view of seclusion: A comparison study," *The Journal of Forensic Psychiatry and Psychology*, 21(3): 446–461.

Latané, B. (1981). "The psychology of social impact," *American Psychologist*, 36(4): 343–356.

Levinas, E. (2006). *Humanism of the Other*, translated by Nidra Poller and Introduction by Richard A. Cohen, Urbana and Chicago: University of Illinois.

Lilja, L. and Hellzén, O. (2008). "Former patients' experiences of psychiatric care: A qualitative investigation," *International Journal of Mental Health Nursing*, 17: 279–286.

Lyon, D. (2007). *Surveillance Studies: An Overview*, Cambridge: Polity Press.

Lyon, D. (2017). "Surveillance culture: Engagement, exposure, and ethics in digital modernity," *International Journal of Communication*, 11: 824–842.

Mann S., Nolan J., and Wellman B. (2003). "Sousveillance: Inventing and using wearable computing devices," *Surveillance and Society*, 1: 331–355.

Marshall, L.A. and Adam, E.A. (2018). "Building from the ground up: Exploring forensic mental staff's relationship with patients," *The Journal of Forensic Psychiatry and Psychology*, 29(5): 744–761.

Marx, G.T. (2003). "A tack in the shoe: Neutralising and resisting new surveillance," *Journal of Social Issues*, 59(2): 369–390.

Marx, G.T. (2009). "A tack in the shoe and taking off the shoe: Neutralisation and counter-neutralisation," *Surveillance and Society*, 6(3): 294–306.

Mathiesen, T. (1997). "The viewer society: Michel Foucault's 'Panopticon' revisited," *Theoretical Criminology*, 1(2): 215–233.

Moore, D. (2011). "The benevolent watch: Therapeutic surveillance in drug treatment court," *Theoretical Criminology*, 15(3): 255–268.

Nail, T. (2017). "What is an assemblage?" *SubStance*, 46(1): 21–37. John Hopkins University Press. Project MUSE Database. Available online: www.muse.jhu.edu [accessed 16 August 2019].

Orwell, G. (1949). *Nineteen Eighty-Four*, London: Secker and Warburg.

Peplau, H.E. (1952). *Interpersonal Relations in Nursing: A Conceptual Frame of Reference for Psychodynamic Nursing*, New York: G.P. Putnam's Sons.

Pinch, T. and Bijker, W.E. (2012). "The social construction of facts and artifacts: or how the sociology of science and the sociology of technology might benefit each other," in Bijker, W.E., Hughes, T.P. and Pinch, T. (eds), *The Social Construction of Technological Systems*, 2nd edition. Cambridge MA: MIT Press 11–45.

Porter, R. (2002). *Madness: A Brief History*, Oxford: Oxford University Press.

Romein, E. and Schuilenburg, M. (2008). "Are you on the fast track? The rise of surveillant assemblages in post-industrial age," *Architectural Theory Review*, 13(3): 337–348.

Rose, N. (1989). *Governing the Soul: The Shaping of the Private Self*, London: Free Association Books.

Ryan, P., Ramon, S. and Greacen, T. (2012). *Empowerment, Lifelong Learning and Recovery in Mental Health*, Basingstoke: Palgrave Macmillan.

Scull, A. (1993). *The Most Solitary of Afflictions*, New Haven: Yale University Press.

Simon, J. (2007). *Governing Through Crime: How the War on Crime Transformed American Democracy and Created a Culture of Fear*, Oxford: Oxford University Press.

Springer, R.A. (2015). "Doing Foucault: Inquiry into nursing knowledge with Foucauldian discourse analysis," *Nursing Philosophy*, 16(2): 87–97.

Staniszewska, S., Mocford, C., Chadburn, G., Fenton, S.-J., Bhui, K., Larkin, M., Newton, E., Crepaz-Keay, D., Griffiths, F. and Weich, S. (2019). "Experiences of in-patient mental health services: Systematic review," *The British Journal of Psychiatry*, 214(6): 329–338.

Stevenson, C. and Cutcliffe, J. (2006). "Problematizing special observation in psychiatry: Foucault, archaeology, genealogy, discourse and power/knowledge," *Journal of Psychiatric Mental Health Nursing*, 13(6): 713–721.

Stevenson, K.N., Jack, S.M., O'Mara, L. and LeGris, J. (2015). "Registered nurses' experiences of patient violence on acute care psychiatric inpatient units: An interpretive descriptive study," *BMC Nursing*, 14(35): 1–13. Available online at https://doi.org/10.1186/s/2912-015-0079-5 [accessed 5 January 2021].

Thompson, N. (2005). *Understanding Social Work: Preparing for Practice*, Basingstoke: Palgrave Macmillan.

Warr, J., Page, M. and Crossen-White, H. (2005). *The Appropriate Use of Closed Circuit Television (CCTV) in a Secure Unit*, Study undertaken by Montpellier Unit and Bournemouth University, England.

Whittington, D. and Ritcher, D. (eds) (2006). *Violence in Mental Health Settings*, New York: Springer.

Wilkie, T., Penney, S.R., Fernane, S. and Simpson, A.I.F. (2014). "Characteristics and motivations of absconders from forensic mental health services: A case-control study," *BMC Psychiatry*, 14(91): 1–13. Available online: https://doi.org/10.1186/1471-244X-14-91 [accessed 23 January 2021].

Yar, M. (2003). "Panoptic power and the pathologisation of vision: Critical reflections on the Foucauldian thesis," *Surveillance and Society*, 1(3): 254–271.

Chapter 3

Implementing CCTV cameras inside mental health wards

Introduction

This chapter provides a background to CCTV implementation. It is not known how many mental health hospitals use CCTV or where the cameras are placed. To establish the extensiveness of camera use inside mental health wards, an audit of all NHS mental health Trusts in England using data gathered from freedom of information legislation was undertaken as part of the research. The research sites included three mental health Trusts in different regions of England. All three wards/units were PICUs. The three PICUs involved in the research were not targeted deliberately; they were included because they were willing to allow access. Similarly, the research sites were also NHS Trusts and not private or independent hospitals. Although private hospitals were approached, they were not willing to participate in the research.

The main body of the chapter is an examination of how each PICU decided to implement CCTV cameras inside it, what ethical concerns they raised, in what ways they expanded surveillance inside the ward and how they have impacted the ward environment. Devolution within the NHS from national to local bodies has resulted in the variation and the reasons for the deployment of CCTV. This has meant that each NHS Trust has individually decided whether they want to use CCTV, which mental health wards require CCTV surveillance, whether the cameras provide recording facilities, live feeds or both, where the cameras should be located, for example, in bedrooms, who should be consulted in the decision-making process, for example, staff, patients and patient groups, how the cameras are reviewed, operated and so on.

Background

Two audits document the use of CCTV inside mental health Trusts and hospitals. The first involved 100 NHS mental health Trusts in England and Wales completed in 2008 (Desai, 2009). The second is an audit undertaken as part of this research completed in 2014 involving 57 NHS mental health Trusts in England only. Both these audits covered all NHS mental health

DOI: 10.4324/9781003179306-3

Table 3.1 Rise in the number of NHS Mental Health Trusts using CCTV

	2008	*2014*
Total number of NHS Mental Health Trusts contacted	100	57
Nil response to FOIA request	29	0
Response to FOIA request	71	57
No. of Trusts with CCTV inside wards	34	36
Approximate number of hospitals with CCTV inside wards	85	128
Approximate number of wards with CCTV	157	388

Trusts at that time. Table 3.1 (below) shows the responses from all the Trusts that were involved in the freedom of information request.

Both audits requested similar information. The Freedom of Information Act 2000 (FOIA) request in 2014 asked for the following information:

- Do you have CCTV cameras located inside any of x (name of NHS Trust) Hospital wards?
- If the answer is yes, can you tell me:
- The name of each Hospital, and the name of the Wards within each Hospital, where CCTV cameras are located on the ward?
- The name of each Hospital, and the name of the Wards within each Hospital, where CCTV cameras are located inside patient bedrooms?
- The name of each Hospital, and the name of Wards within each Hospital, where CCTV cameras are located inside seclusion rooms?

These audits suggest that in the six years between 2008 and 2014, there has been an approximate 147 per cent increase in the number of wards using CCTV. This roughly equates to a 25 per cent rise each year in the number of mental health wards choosing to implement CCTV inside them. The average number of communal area cameras (excluding bedroom cameras) used inside the three mental health wards, which were part of this study, equated to 10 cameras. This figure, when multiplied by 388 wards using CCTV cameras, suggests that there are approximately over 3,880 cameras deployed in communal areas inside mental health wards in England. These figures give an approximation and do not reveal the full scale of CCTV use as they do not cover private or independent hospitals. The FOIA 2000 only extends to the public sector, and private hospitals are not obliged to be transparent about this information. Hence, the total number of hospitals and wards using CCTV is likely to be higher. However, what these figures do confirm is that the use of CCTV is not diminishing and is on the rise.

Tully et al. (2016) believe that CCTV cameras have featured as a surveillance tool inside high-security mental hospitals since 2002. Despite the rise in the use of CCTV cameras inside mental health wards, there is no specific national policy or political event that has resulted in a push for the need for cameras inside it. Therefore, the narrative of how the cameras have found their way from managing security around the periphery of the hospital to inside the mental health ward including patient bedrooms is missing. Similarly, there is no specific policy, nationally or locally within mental health Trusts, as to how the cameras should be used inside the ward. As a result, camera uses inside the ward have evolved where some of these uses have retrospectively been included in guidance documents (DH, 2013; NAPICU, 2014; NAPICU, 2017). The lack of clarity in the use of CCTV cameras inside the ward is also apparent in the inconsistency of guidance provided by these documents. For example, NAPICU (2014) guidance encourages the use of infrared cameras and audio equipment in the monitoring of patients in their bedroom at night time, while the Department of Health (2013) guidance suggests that CCTV cameras should not be used inside patient bedrooms. This lack of attention to the growing use of cameras in the ward was reflected in the decisions made to implement cameras inside each research site PICU.

The three research sites and location of CCTV cameras

Site 1

Site 1 is a relatively new, purpose-built PICU. It is the first ward within the Trust to use CCTV camera technology inside it. CCTV cameras were located in air-locked spaces, visitor room, seclusion room, a de-escalation room (similar in design to a seclusion room where patients are segregated for a short time from for observation), garden areas and exits. There were two CCTV monitors in the ward office, which were visible to patients. Staff were aware that patients could view the CCTV monitors, and during most of the fieldwork observations inside site 1, the blinds on the window adjoining the ward remained shut so that patients were restricted in their ability to view these monitors. There was no dedicated staff whose job it was to watch the monitors. However, most permanent staff did use the cameras, and they were able to change the screens on the monitors, for example, to enlarge it, reduce it or switch it off. There were two further monitors, one in the seclusion lobby (adjoining the seclusion room) that allowed staff to watch patients in seclusion using CCTV, and one in the de-escalation lobby (adjoining the de-escalation room) that allowed staff to watch patients in the de-escalation room using CCTV. The cameras in the seclusion room and the de-escalation room also provided a live feed to the ward office monitors. All CCTV cameras inside site 1 did not record and provided live feeds only.

Of the three case study sites, site 1 is the only Trust that decided to use live feeds only. Managers emphasised the tension in taking the decision not to record CCTV footage. Their concerns for not recording CCTV footage were primarily linked to implications concerning the 1998 Data Protection Act and the added requirements that the legislation entails concerning the storage, safety and security of recorded materials. However, it was not solely limited to this, and managers also described other aspects such as the potential for CCTV to erode patient privacy. Yet despite this concern, their primary reason for having the cameras in the ward was to "have more eyes about the place" (comment made by a manager, M1), so that staff would always know the whereabouts of patients inside it. Privacy in this respect was limited to not using CCTV in what managers described as "private" spaces inside the ward; these spaces included patient bedrooms, bathrooms and toilets.

Site 2

Site 2 has been open for the longest length of time of the three sites. It was a refurbished ward and was located in an older building that has several difficult-to-observe areas or blind-spots. At the commencement of fieldwork observations, CCTV cameras were located in air-locked space, activity room, the female sitting area located at the end of the female ward, inside the original entrance to the building located at the end of the male ward area, which could also be used as a de-escalation area, garden area and television lounge area. There were two CCTV monitors located inside the ward. The monitor located in the ward office could easily be seen by patients in the ward. During research fieldwork observations, several patients were observed looking intently at the monitor. There was no dedicated staff to watch the monitors. The staff could not change the screen settings from the ward office. There was a further CCTV monitor located in the ward manager's office. The ward manager and some senior nursing staff had access to this facility. The cameras provided a live feed and recording facility, and screen settings could only be changed via the monitor in the ward manager's office.

Of the three sites, site 2 has had cameras inside the ward for the longest time including having more cameras in what are communal parts of the ward, such as the television lounge area and activity room. It was difficult to decipher what the original reasons were for installing CCTV other than at that time the clinical team felt that it was needed. Similarly, site 2 originally had a seclusion room inside it; however, this facility no longer exists in the ward. Other than the de-escalation space at the end of the male corridor, this site had no other dedicated suite of rooms where they could isolate a patient, from other patients and staff. During the majority of research fieldwork observation inside this site, CCTV cameras were operating mainly on live feed only. The cameras did have the ability to record, but this facility was only working sporadically because there had been no upkeep and regular maintenance of the cameras. Towards the end of the fieldwork observation period, existing cameras were replaced from analogue to digital, and additional cameras were added. The decision to replace and add new cameras was taken before the commencement of the research. Managers at site 2 identified the rationale for the additional cameras as:

- Providing evidence for any incident that happens in the ward, especially where there is a serious assault and the case has to be taken to court.
- As a learning tool for any incident that occurs as a way of reviewing practices and enabling a debrief process.
- To cover difficult to supervise areas inside the ward and the courtyard area.

The consequence of additional cameras in the ward meant that cameras covering the lounge and dining area, for example, increased from one camera in this area to three. The cameras were also introduced around all communal spaces and patient corridors in the ward which previously were not covered.

Site 3

Site 3 is a relatively new unit. It was a purpose-built PICU. CCTV cameras were located in air-locked space, entrance covering female ward, entrance to visitor's room from the ward, entrance inside the main ward, female communal area, visitor's room, garden areas and Extra-Care Area (which, inside this PICU, was a suite of rooms designed the same as seclusion facilities) used for de-escalation of patients. While separate sleeping areas for women were apparent in all three sites, site 3 was the only site that also used additional cameras in the female corridor area and similar to site 2 in the female lounge area. The female corridor was only accessible via a specially programmed key fob, which was allocated to female patients and staff. Hence, male patients could not enter this area as their key fob would not have allowed them access. The placement of cameras in the female area of the ward created a specific gender dimension to camera placement, discussed in more detail later in this and other chapters.

The ward also used infrared cameras and audio equipment located individually in each patient bedroom for less disruptive night-time observations. According to managers, these cameras were only used for those patients who had consented to be monitored in this way. Bedroom cameras provided live feeds only and were only operational when staff were undertaking patient observations in this way. There were two CCTV monitors in the ward office which were partially visible to patients. There was no dedicated staff whose job it was to watch CCTV monitors. However, most permanent staff knew how to change screen settings from the ward office. The cameras in the Extra-Care Area and communal areas provided a live feed and recording facility.

Site 3 also decided to include an infrared CCTV camera and audio equipment inside each patient bedroom when the PICU was relocated to the new purpose-built site. Managers at site 3 identified the reasons for the cameras in communal areas as:

- Providing additional observations in the courtyard area where it can be difficult to supervise patients.
- Providing additional cover to certain areas in the ward such as the entrance to the female ward for the safety of female patients.
- Providing additional evidence in the event of a serious incident on the ward either to investigate the incident for the Trust or as evidence in any court hearing.
- For training and review of practice.

Site 3 also had several cameras outside the PICU entrance. These cameras were used to:

- Monitor people coming to the unit.
- Provide an up-to-date picture of any patient who has absconded from the unit to the police as a missing person.
- Monitor patients at the front of the building as part of their leave arrangement (explained in more detail in Chapter 4). Table 3.2 (below) identifies camera locations inside all three PICUs.

Table 3.2 Location of cameras and CCTV monitors in all three sites

Spaces inside the ward	*Site 1*	*Site 2*	*Site 3*
Air-locked space	√	√	√
Visitor room	√	x	√
Seclusion room	√	x	x
De-escalation room/extra-care area	√	√	√
Garden/courtyard area	√	√	√
Exit door from the ward	x	√	√
Activity room	x	√	x
Lounge area	x	√	x
Female ward entrance area	x	√	√
Male ward entrance area	√	x	x
Infrared night-time cameras inside patient bedrooms	x	x	√
Ward office area	x	√	x
Dining area	x	√	x
Recording facility	x	√	√
Live feed only	√	x	x
CCTV monitor in ward office	√	√	√
CCTV monitor in manager office	x	√	x
CCTV monitor in seclusion lobby	√	x	x
CCTV monitor in de-escalation/extra-care area	√	x	x

Drivers for CCTV use

Fixing problems

Some managers agreed that there is very little research or evidence related to the benefits of using CCTV inside mental health wards. However, these managers felt that the ability of the cameras to do basic tasks, such as opening up spaces inside the ward, made them a useful tool. The addition of cameras inside sites 1 and 3 came about as a result of specific individuals who were interested in implementing cameras.

> M3: *"We had a Director of Nursing … I must be going back 15 years at least … he started the conversations about CCTV …"*

The final decision to include cameras inside the ward was a local one. In addition to particular individuals who pushed for cameras inside the ward, the decision to implement cameras was also influenced by several other factors. Below, for example, M6 describes how an incident inside his own mental health Trust resulted in the addition of more cameras, including a change in system from analogue to digital recording.

> M6: *"… and that we needed to put in extra cameras cos there was blind spots that came about because we had erm an incident where a member of staff broke their leg in a … restraint situation but the CCTV didn't pick it up".*

A few managers did not necessarily believe that implementing cameras or having more cameras in the ward would resolve problems. They perceived the implementation of cameras as a "knee-jerk" response, based on quick-fix solutions. These incidents do not have to occur inside their own hospital or NHS Trust, and for these managers, the cameras were perceived as an easy solution by those in authority.

> M7: *"I think in my role one of the single criticisms that I have of most of the jobs we do is that we don't actually know what we want … Whereas if we spent a little bit more time about right what is it, whether I'm building a new hospital, whether I'm refurbishing a ward or whether I'm installing a new CCTV system what is the desired outcome …"*

This lack of focus and response to incidents are not unusual within the NHS. For example, South West London and St George's Mental Health Trust placed CCTV cameras monitored by security guards inside its intensive care ward after it was fined £28,000 for pleading guilty to the murder of a healthcare assistant by a patient (Laurance, 2005). The Trust, following an internal review, eventually abandoned the use of security staff in monitoring the cameras (Chambers and Gillard, 2005). As McCahill (2012: 247) states, this form of synoptic representation, in this instance, the negligence of care from a known and dangerous patient, generates support for "further panoptic measures". Monahan (2011: 496) cautions against perceiving technologies "as exogenous tools", which are mobilised "to deal with perceived problems or needs". He asserts the importance of viewing technologies in the context of cultural practices and social systems where the cameras are examined as agents or actants within that system. Most managers believed that the appeal of the cameras inside the ward was predominantly based on their perceived ability to resolve problems in the ward and not always their actual ability to do this.

When deciding to implement CCTV, managers also spoke of being prepared for any changes in government directive or policy as a result of a knee-jerk response to an incident that could become a national issue. These managers spoke about implementing the cameras as part of "future-proofing" the ward in the event of a potential incident that may lead to a national crisis. The implementation of the cameras was therefore designed around an event that may or may not happen but where managers believed that they were ready to respond should the need arise.

> M2: *"... there's a mixture of opinion but there's a good chance if we want it in the future, we don't exactly know how we'll use it but let's just build it in because why would you not do it and have to go back and put it in. It's so disruptive isn't it, so let's just you know go with a fairly minimum thing put it in and then deal with it after and the worst-case scenario if you don't want to use it, then don't use it".*

It was therefore the threat of the politicisation of a potential incident in the future which was used as a driver to implement the cameras inside the ward, thus supporting Deleuze and Gautarri's (1980) claim that assemblages are political. Site 1 choose to implement CCTV and limited its use to live feed only where some managers believed that the full capacity of the cameras could be deployed should it be necessary.

No limits to camera use

The rhizomatic nature of surveillance, as described by Deleuze and Guattari (1980), was apparent in the desire to use the cameras to up open more flows and spaces of control. Below, M5 sums up the views of several managers who believed that not drawing on the (yet unknown) full potential of the cameras constituted a missed opportunity.

> M5: *"We should look at using the system [CCTV] for all sorts of different purposes and that, that's my feeling on it. It is not just, shouldn't just be used for any one sole purpose. It's there, you've got a system ... that you can do all sorts of elements with ..."*

In an ever-increasing busy world where managers are expected to be in several different places and several different locations, camera expansion was also viewed by some as a way of keeping an eye on the ward when they were not inside it. This was the case even for those managers who did not have clinical responsibility inside the ward. The capability of the cameras to open up ward spaces through the ability to look back at recordings meant that managers believed that they could stay connected with the ward at all times. This allowed managers to permeate the ward environment in a way that was not possible before. In this way, the modern mental health hospital also stands apart from asylum care which was defined by its limited permeability where movement in and out of the asylum was limited by its size and location.

> M8: *"... we can access the rest of the hospital's cameras from a computer here via the software ... and the reason for this is that out-of-hours because we tend to have one extra member of staff on nights here, so the wards come to us. For example, if the police need an image of somebody who's absconded from the hospital in the night, we can access that and provide that via remote location on a lap-top here".*
>
> M10: *"... what I'm trying to do is we're taking all the information, we're taking all the CCTV and upgrading them ... it means that I can literally, on my lap-top now, here, or at home, should there be an incident, or should there be someone gone missing, where we now have digital cameras linked up to the Trust network, I can dial in from home. If the police want a picture of, you know, Joe Bloggs at two in the morning, someone can give me a call. I can dial into that system. If I know that he left at 1.15 in the morning or thereabouts. I can search and take a snapshot picture within minutes. I can email that to the police, so yeah, I can dial into about five locations currently".*
>
> M6: *"So in an ideal world ... I'd like to have, be able to tap in and have access to all the CCTV around the Trust ... have it all linked to one computer back at head office that'd be ideal".*

Societal expectations

The impervious nature of asylums not only related to their physical presence, but the nature of patient care inside them meant they were also cut off from society. PICUs stand apart from this, and while they were physically difficult to access or leave, they are still linked to the outside world in several ways. For example, most patients inside all three research sites were allowed visitors, and although there were set times for visits, these were not always adhered to explicitly. Patients woke up when they wanted, went to bed when they wanted, participated in ward activities or occupational therapy activities, sometimes away from the ward. In addition, some patients had approved leave to walk around or sit outside the PICU, others had approved leave and had accompanied walks with staff to the shops, some PICUs allowed some patients to have their mobile phone or have access to their phone and so on. Most managers recognised that these activities came with risks, for instance, the risk of a patient or their visitor bringing weapons, alcohol or other banned substances or items into the ward. The cameras were perceived as a measure to allow the flow of activities inside the ward while managing these risks. However, these risks were not only linked to the behaviour of patients but also the type of patients that were inside them. All three research sites cared for patients who were acutely ill, some patients were also thought to have consumed or had an addiction to illegal substances, some were angry about being detained, some were bored, some were frightened, some harboured thoughts about hurting themselves, some worried that they would not be discharged and so forth. These factors also made patients inside the PICU a risk, therefore, managers believed that it would be a given that cameras should also be inside the ward. M7 (below) surmises how the cameras found their way inside his PICU:

> M7: *"So, for instance, when it came to CCTV I would, I would bet my bottom dollar that started off with and of course we're going to need CCTV ... it's a mental health unit, therefore, it will have CCTV".*
>
> M9: *"The expectation that stuff happening will somehow be recorded in one way or another has become by osmosis in many ways expected ... and I've certainly been involved in scenarios where stuff's happened and there's been an expectation, well there'll be CCTV of that, won't there".*

In this way, communal area cameras were not perceived by managers as apparatus that needed any additional attention. Their arrival inside the ward was considered alongside a range of other technological innovations related to monitoring behaviour as M9 (below) explains.

> M9: *"so we got computer notes now, every fob when you came in here and the fob I touched on the door is all auditable ... sometimes you're even checked down to the extent of lateness or attendance or non-attendance".*

The belief that society, staff, patients and their visitors would expect PICUs to have cameras also influenced who held responsibility for the cameras. Across all three Trusts, managers identified a range of other managers whom they believed were responsible for the cameras. These included the ward manager, security officer, Chief Executive of the Trust, in-patient directorate and estates as having primary responsibility. An outcome of this was that staff and patients were unsure about who they should approach if they had concerns about the cameras. Below, two staff – S14 and S23 – were surprised that they could not do anything about the cameras.

> S14: *"I don't think there's anything that I could do, is there? I don't know".*
>
> S23: *"I don't think I would go to a manager and say I don't like the cameras watching me".*

The expectation that the cameras are a part of the ward similar to other safety features, such as personal alarms, locked wards and so on, meant that most managers generally worked on the assumption that staff and patients were satisfied with the cameras. They made this assumption on the basis that they had not received any complaints about them.

> M2: *"I guess the fact we haven't had any, we've had no complaints relating to it at all … So I guess that suggests its, well there's nothing immediately alarming about it … or we would have heard about it …"*
>
> M5: *"Erm none of the staff have ever come out and opposed, it's been raised at various meetings".*

Therefore, several managers assumed that the presence of cameras in society normalised the presence of cameras inside the ward. They did not expect patients or staff to be disturbed by the cameras which they believed linked the ward to wider society. These managers believed that CCTV cameras are to be found everywhere and are mostly accepted by society. Webster (2009) highlights how people's perceptions of the technological capabilities of CCTV influence their decision-making. He suggests that this is the case even though there is sometimes no evidence to suggest that the cameras actually work for the task that they were initially deployed, which inside the mental health ward was not always very clear.

Patient and staff involvement in the decision to implement CCTV

CCTV in communal areas

Whereas asylums regarded patients as docile bodies that were voiceless, modern mental health hospitals encourage patients to voice their opinion and become active participants in how care is delivered. Jørgensen and Rendtorff (2017) describe how patient participation has become the key goal in mental health care, where some hospitals also encourage staff to refer to patients as clients or service users. These terms were used by staff in the research sites as a way of acknowledging patients as active recipients of care, albeit that these patients were detained in hospital and therefore not voluntary service users. In an organisational context, patients are also described as stakeholders. In their role as stakeholders, they are encouraged to actively participate in the development and functioning of the hospital. The mental health hospital, therefore, actively seeks out patient views as a means of improving their plans and delivery of health care. In the three case study sites, managers described how patient views on installing or expanding CCTV in communal areas were garnered.

> M1: "*... when we designed the ward ... we involved service users and staff ... We did involve service users as part of ... asking the question about should we be using CCTV*".
>
> M3: "*I don't remember whether we surveyed staff but I certainly remember we had a meeting here with service users input, estates input and some of the clinical staff, and we debated all the fors and against, and we did, we did a kind of erm, well we captured all the reasons why*".
>
> M5: "*As far as patients are concerned the interaction has been very much, we're looking to do this work and we try and consult at different times with patients around what it is we're looking at. So whether that's furniture, or whether that's changes to the environment, or plans for future activity, plans for future change, we always try and capture that from the individuals [patients] that are there [on the ward] at the time*".
>
> M9: "*so in the different meetings we had, we had a planning committee ... for most of it, a range of disciplines that work here, a service user representative ... and then we had the estates people ... and what they call the M and E people, mechanical and electrical ...*"

Although patients and staff were invited to participate in the decision to implement CCTV, it was less clear how their views influenced any outcomes. Some managers, for example, were not always able to fully explain what issues patients had raised about CCTV implementation inside the ward.

> M2: "*I think getting a service user view that's balanced is a challenge as well. Like we had polar in the room, you know, somebody that's totally adamant, don't you dare put it in, it's awful. And somebody else, oh yeah put it everywhere and keep me safe and you think they're both equally valid*".
>
> M3: "*I can't remember it [CCTV] being on the wish-list [staff wish-list]. I don't remember seeing it on there. It was certainly one of those early discussions about future-proof, and there were lots of people saying that we don't want it in this kind of environment, and a small group saying we do*".

Therefore, in principle, patients and staff can give their views and raise any concerns about whether they want CCTV cameras within communal areas of the ward. However, the fact that managers had already decided that the ward would implement the cameras meant that their views remained as opinions only.

CCTV in bedrooms

Site 3 chose to implement infrared CCTV and audio equipment inside patient bedrooms to undertake night-time nursing observations of patients. This decision was primarily influenced by the availability of technology as a problem-solver and an enabler.

> M9: *"The use of CCTV as a piece of equipment, by which I mean the ability to see where otherwise couldn't be seen ... with an audit trail. I don't mean in the images, but I mean in the fact that a look was made, the basis of that was very straightforward, erm additional option to meet a commonly reported problem in a mental health setting. So put simply, a technological solution to a problem presented itself, mostly for patients, and that was for a period of less disturbance during night-time sleeping hours".*

While some managers extolled the benefits of CCTV for undertaking nurse observation practices that are less disruptive at night time, other managers, especially in sites 1 and 2, believed that bedrooms were private spaces and should not be open to CCTV surveillance. However, what is deemed as a private space and public space in the context of the ward is difficult to decipher. Below, a manager from site 2 explains how camera placement was avoided in patient bedrooms in order to maintain patient dignity.

> M5: *"... camera settings has been taken into consideration because of elements with regard to where the cameras are looking ... obviously we want to avoid, avoid the privacy and dignity of bedrooms and various other places".*

However, it can be argued that any space where it is not possible to see patients at all times is an unsafe space, including bedrooms and toilets. The use of cameras inside toilets was considered to be inappropriate by most managers. However, the use of cameras inside toilets is not new. Taylor (2010), for example, highlights the use of CCTV cameras inside toilets in schools. Inside the ward, patients can arguably harm themselves, or be harmed by others, inside their bedroom and toilets in the same way that they can inside communal areas of the ward. They are also monitored inside their bedroom to ensure their safety. However, the majority of managers, staff and patients did not like the idea of cameras being in what they described as private spaces of the ward, namely bedrooms and toilets. The decision-making concerning camera implementation in what several managers considered as private spaces of the ward, therefore, remained arbitrary.

The ethical principle of privacy and dignity of patients and the use of CCTV inside bedrooms is complex. The reality is that patients do not have a choice about whether they are observed inside their bedroom or not. Even though they may not be a suicide risk, all patients are observed (through nurse observations) at the same time intervals (that is, every hour or 30 minutes) throughout the night as they are during the day. Individual patients may be subject to higher levels of observation, dependent on their risk level and propensity to harm themselves or harm others. Macnish (2014) raises the question of proportionality in relation to surveillance, an issue which, in relation to privacy, has been established in human rights legislation and often cited in the context of the mental health ward. Article 8 of the Human Rights Act 1998 claims that people have a right to a private and family life. The Act goes on to say that any limitations to this must be covered by law, that it should be necessary and proportionate, and it should be for one or more of the following aims:

- Public safety or the country's economic well-being;
- Prevention of disorder or crime;
- Protecting health or morals;
- Protecting other people's rights and freedoms;
- National security.

What is proportionate in law has yet to be fully established because there has been no legal challenge around privacy and the use of CCTV cameras inside mental health wards. In applying the principle of proportionality, it could be argued that when patients are in their bedroom, their risk, unless that patient is suicidal, is reduced. This is because the likelihood of them being harmed by others or them harming others is reduced. However, risk management does not happen in this way. Patients are considered to be at the same risk levels during the night as they are throughout the day. Beck (1992) characterises modern society as a "risk society" which Giddens (1998) claims is preoccupied not only with future risk minimisation but also with safety. It is this notion of keeping patients safe at all times, including at night, when they are not at risk of harm from other patients, which promotes their additional surveillance. Below, M9 describes the pressures that managers are under in maintaining the safety of patients even though sometimes this is at the detriment of patient welfare.

> M9: *"Separate debate but nevertheless, in developed democracies, I suppose in which people have their expectations of care and consideration. People just don't, they won't sit very well with the idea in psychiatric intensive care unit. For example, somebody [patient] went to bed at 9, they died at 11 at night but we wouldn't know about it until we open the door at 9 in the morning. People just won't accept that as due care and attention for a facility of this type, so interval observation has become, err it's become a procedure to deal with that problem".*

Several managers at site 3 perceived CCTV inside bedrooms as a way of seeking a solution for this problem. They saw CCTV as a benefit in enabling them to resolve or at least provide patients with an option, to use the cameras as a way of undertaking discrete monitoring so they can have the benefit of uninterrupted sleep. It is possibly because CCTV camera use inside patient bedroom would directly affect patients that when implementing cameras and audio equipment inside bedrooms, site 3 made the most effort in proactively seeking patient and staff views about the system. A mock-up of the technology was set up between two offices so that patients and staff could see how the system would work.

> M9: *"The way we tested the … function and the technology for the night-time observation system we had one set up here, looking into the office next door. So … we had hordes of people come through here … at one point err I think probably 40 or 50 people, groups of service users [patients] come in to see it … but that was all part of it really, how it worked, the system, the all-in system … each person had to fill out a semi-structured thing [form] about what they thought about the system and so on".*
>
> M8: *"We were talked to by M9 and I think Dr. X was as well … it was a mock system that had been set up from M9's office to Dr. X's office … the plan was to show the clinicians and canvass the views really on whether the system should be, should it record erm people [patients] that have been there, should it immediately upload to the observation profiles on the clinical system? You know, should it be a recording camera system in the patient's room but I think we moved, that was moved away from on the basis of ethics really because having a recorded CCTV … wasn't the purpose of the system, the purpose of the system was purely to help patients have a good night's sleep and I think that premise was stuck to".*

Patients were encouraged to contribute to how the cameras would operate and be used. However, this way of engaging patients in surveillance technologies inside the ward gives them limited choices. The participation of the patient in decision-making is based on their understanding that medical power inside the ward is based on their ability to give themselves over to the medical gaze. These social relations impact how views and opinions are sought inside the ward, and ideally, as Kelly (2009) argues, this multi-directionality of power does not only have to flow from the powerful to the powerless but also can flow from below simultaneously. However, patients did not have a choice as to whether their bedroom has a camera in it or not; their choice was limited to how the cameras were used. For example, any patient who did not want to be monitored by bedroom cameras can refuse to give their consent. These patients, however, would still be subject to an in-person check, where this in-person check would require a staff member to shine a torch through a glass panel located on the bedroom door and, if it were not possible to view the patient clearly, to enter the bedroom and switch on the night light so that staff could reassure themselves that the patient was still alive. Alternatively, the choice was to give consent to the use of infrared cameras and audio equipment to carry out the same activity but with minimum disruption. In this way, patient and staff views of bedroom cameras were limited to their functionality where the fundamental decision as to whether the cameras should be inside bedrooms or not had already been made by managers.

Privacy and dignity

Most managers paid little attention to how staff used the cameras in their day-to-day activities inside the PICU. As the next chapter goes on to discuss this is primarily because inside all three research sites there were no standard operating procedures on how communal area cameras should be used. Therefore, institutional audits of the cameras undertaken by the hospital such as privacy impact assessments tended to uphold the rights of the public. Below, M10 describes how cameras were viewed by most managers in all three research sites where the driver for camera use inside the PICU differed to their use from the cameras based around the periphery of the hospital.

> M10: *"Privacy impact assessment I would really apply to external cameras, obviously we don't want to be prying or catching, you know accidentally somebody's lounge windows err we don't want that sort of thing … the internal side of it I'd be suggesting that we're going to replace camera, camera 1 that may look at the communal areas, how many incidents of violence and aggression have taken place in that area, do we need it?"*

Therefore, managers responsible for privacy impact audits were more concerned about undermining the privacy of the public, over patients. According to M10 (above), internal audits of cameras are about the number of incidents inside the ward, which have not been captured on camera. This is because privacy inside the ward is regarded as a qualified right, which means that a person's rights are limited because they have to be balanced with the interests of other patients, staff and organisational requirements. For example, a patient who seeks to harm himself or herself inside the ward cannot have an absolute right to privacy. Therefore, Stolovy et al. (2015: 276) claim that ward spaces are not private spaces; they are public spaces and that public spaces in the ward also include patient bedrooms, where patients need to be monitored because they have the opportunity to harm themselves. Marx (2001) argues that discussions around the concept of privacy are often ambiguous. He suggests that the meaning of what is public or private space is in the interpretation and meaning of how aspects such as CCTV are interpreted and framed. Gilligan (1982) argues that traditional ethical theories about privacy are based on legal frameworks which suggest that they are universal and impartial views and that any intrusion of privacy inside the ward is justifiable on the basis that it can potentially deter violence, criminal behaviour and harm to patients and is done for the common good.

Some managers tended to prioritise privacy inside the ward with maintaining patient dignity. Their interpretation of privacy primarily focused on pragmatic concerns, including ensuring that the cameras were not capturing patients in potentially undignified situations.

> M2: *"We haven't put it [CCTV] in the en-suite seclusion room ... we had a bit of a discussion about that, so we've kept with having viewing panels and not cameras ... I think when we've had discussions about that ... If it's a woman and it's a male member of staff ... it just feels to me, you know, if you're having a shower in there, and the thought of a camera in there. It feels a step too far. Although probably somebody would be able to open the window and still look at you. It's difficult, isn't it? But it feels like a different level of concern really".*

Lyon (1994) argues that rather than reducing privacy debates about CCTV to the technical or legal, it makes more sense to see it as a social relation. For example, taking into account M2's concerns (in the quote above), there is a difference between watching a female patient taking a shower using a camera and watching her face-to-face. This is because the face-to-face encounter changes the nature of looking into a social relation. The staff member looking has to confront his feelings about looking at the female patient's naked body. Similarly, the female patient can also see the male staff looking at her. It is in this way that watching a patient face-to-face is different. When using a CCTV camera to watch a patient in this way, not only does the patient not know who is looking at them, but also how long they have spent looking at them in this way.

Goffman (1969) uses the terms "front stage" and "back stage" to refer to the different behaviours that people engage in everyday life. He suggests that social life is a performance carried out by people in three places; these include "front stage", "back stage" and "off stage" behaviours. His dramaturgical analysis is used as a means of understanding human interactions. Inside the ward, as well as staff, patients can also behave in different ways according to where they are. During fieldwork observations, several patients explained that they made themselves enter communal areas of the ward, even though they did not enjoy being around other people. This was one of the ways that patients believed that they could demonstrate to staff that they were well enough to be discharged from the ward. Similarly, those patients who had cameras inside their bedroom did not believe that staff would not be interested in their back stage behaviour as a means of assessing their wellness. Therefore, these patients did not always believe that staff would not use cameras to look at them outside observation times (see Chapter 5). Warr et al. (2005) have already shown how easy it is to use the cameras for a different purpose (see Chapter 2). Although the bedroom camera set up inside site 3 was different to bedroom camera set up in Warr et al.'s study, in that staff could not access the cameras from the ward office, not all patients believed this. Unlike communal areas where there were no standard operating procedures related to camera use, this was not the case with bedroom camera use. In this way, bedroom camera use was much more restricted. For example, bedroom cameras could only be operated by staff between 10 p.m. and 7 a.m.

Although the bedroom may provide a sanctuary for patients from having to perform for staff in communal areas of the ward, this was not the case for patients inside seclusion. Seclusion is used as containment where the disciplinary power of seclusion is in the knowledge that one is seen continuously. Inside seclusion, there are very limited spaces for back stage and off stage behaviour because the patient knows that they are seen all the time, including when they are showering or using the toilet. During fieldwork observations, few patients spent a long time inside the shower and toilet where there were no cameras, whilst some often used a blanket to cover their body possibly to gain relief from being constantly looked at. This can be difficult for patients as they struggle to maintain privacy between front stage and back stage behaviour, and as the next chapter goes on to discuss, it also impacted how staff interpreted this behaviour.

CCTV in female ward areas: Gendered surveillance

Sites 1 and 3 had locked access to female-only ward areas. On site 3, female patients had their own key fobs which allowed them access inside this ward area. Both these sites also had a specifically designated locked lounge area for those women who preferred to stay away from male patients. It was possible on all three sites to physically see the ward entrance to the female ward area from the ward office. Site 3 not only had visible access to the female ward area, it also had two cameras monitoring the female ward area. One camera was located at the entrance to the female ward area, and the other was located inside the female communal area, which had seating and a television set. This camera could view not only the communal area but also two of the three female-only bedrooms located in this area. This meant that women patients could be seen on CCTV the moment they left their bedroom.

A recent examination of sexual incidents inside mental health wards by the Care Quality Commission (September 2018) between April and June 2017 suggested that of the 60,000 incidents recorded during this period, 298 incidents involved nakedness or exposure, 273 included sexual assaults, 242 included using verbal abuse using sexual words, 184 incidents of sexual harassment and 29 allegations of rape, with women most likely to be affected. Most of these incidents were thought to have taken place within communal areas of the ward (416 incidents), with smaller numbers inside patient bedrooms or other areas such as toilets and bathrooms (194 incidents) and in garden and courtyard areas (70 incidents) and in areas where staff would be present (23 incidents). These figures suggest that it is not necessarily private spaces inside the ward where patients are vulnerable; it is the communal areas and those spaces that are monitored by staff. The visibility of spaces and the exposure of women patient bodies, therefore, do not necessarily result in making women patients safer inside the ward.

The exposure of violence inside mental health hospitals since the early 1990s has highlighted the specific abuse experienced by women patients inside wards. Perhaps one of the most influential documents which raised concern around women's mental health was the Department of Health's (September 2002) "*Women's Mental Health: Into the Mainstream*". This document called for a more gendered approach to mental health care which recognises a range of socio-economic, physiological and psychological factors associated with women's mental health. For example, factors such as, "women's mental health is affected by experiences of child sexual abuse, domestic violence, sexual violence and rape" (DH, September 2002: 12). Inside some wards, women's fundamental right to be kept safe has been interpreted by managers as the need to protect them by increasing their surveillance. Koskela (2012) believes that women as targets of surveillance are gendered in at least three senses, and this includes how the need to protect them is perceived. Below, M9 describes how the decision to place cameras inside the female lounge area and at the entrance of the female ward area was influenced:

> M9: *"So mixed gender PICUs present particular problems. The female service user lobby is quite strong in this, and I'm sure you've come across it, people [female patients] often feel frightened, sexually harassed, or abused or in times when they're making not the best judgements, potentially vulnerable. Because we've got a mixed gender thing [ward], we've got other electronic protections like the female fob will only open the female area, and the male fob will only open the male area. And there is a separation by a staff basis, you will have seen and there's one interchangeable bed on the other side of the staff base. So, the approach to the female area is covered by CCTV, so if someone was to take somebody into the female area or somebody was attempting to get into it, we would be able to evidence back who that was. Erm so that's why we put it there".*

Therefore, CCTV cameras place women as victims of usually male violence under more surveillance. Koskela (2012) draws on feminist literature to highlight the exposure of women's bodies, which, she claims, is viewed differently from male bodies. As part of their ethical consideration in relation to deciding whether to place cameras in the female lounge area or not, M8 (below) describes how women's bodies are exposed the moment they enter the communal area:

> M8: *"Yeah I mean ... there were huge ethical consideration around, again particularly the female area because not only, again there's another balance isn't there, protecting females but then absolutely acknowledging that if a female does come out of her room naked they're actually on camera. So there's another sort of example of erm and how are they going to feel, if they're better and they realise that that's the case ... yeah I am aware that was all considered relatively, erm well not relatively, strongly and obviously a balance reached really in terms of what we implemented".*

Inside the ward, women not only have to accept more surveillance, but they also have to recognise that this surveillance is not necessarily going to stop them from being attacked by male patients or staff. This is because as M9 (above) has described CCTV use in those PICUs that have recording facility often happens retrospectively. Hence, it is only when an allegation is made, or a concern has been raised, that staff can look back at CCTV footage to determine whether it is true or false. Therefore, the cameras do not protect women patients in real-time, where women patients also have to accept that their bodies will be exposed to more surveillance at a time when they are not always in a position to control their behaviour. In this respect, the onus placed on women to pay attention to how they are seen is not negated because of their mental health condition (Koskela, 2012).

CCTV in communal areas

Blind-spots and hot-spots

Similar to bedroom cameras, the decision to use CCTV in communal areas of the ward was also driven by the availability of the technology. However, the placement of cameras in communal areas of the ward was not influenced by the number of violent incidents that happened in those areas of the ward. For example, during fieldwork observations inside all three wards, the areas where patients tended to become most agitated was around the ward office entrance and corridor spaces near the ward office. Regardless of the number of staff available in communal areas of the ward, patients tended to want attention from staff in the office. This was possibly because some patients recognised that the qualified nursing staff, who were more able to meet their demands, tended to stay inside the ward office doing administration tasks. Patients also came to the ward office to gain access to their cigarettes, money or to find out when they could go on leave, or when they could see their psychiatrist, and so on. It is usually around the ward office entrance that patients might be denied access to items, or be told that they cannot go on leave, or meet with their psychiatrist at that moment, and it was often these encounters that led to aggression in those areas of the ward. This was also the case in the dining areas of wards. During meal times, all patients congregated in the dining area at the same time, and this occasionally led to patients becoming irritated with one another as they were less tolerant of other patient's behaviours. Inside all three PICUs, patients generally had one hot meal each day, and therefore these meal times were important to them. This meant that some areas in the ward, such as the area immediately outside the ward office and dining room area, became "hot-spots" for disruptive and sometimes aggressive behaviour. These hot-spot areas were a source of animosity between some staff and managers (discussed again in Chapter 4).

Camera placements were generally justified by managers on the basis that they covered areas that were difficult to supervise (or blind-spots). Managers also emphasised that in blind-spot areas (where the cameras had the capacity for recording), CCTV footage was generally used retrospectively. The preferred option by managers to implement cameras inside blind-spot areas of the ward and not the hot-spot areas highlighted two significant concerns. First, because the cameras simultaneously acted as a tool for deterrence and evidence gathering; it meant that their placement inside the ward would always remain contentious. This was because most patient aggression did not happen in blind-spot areas of the ward but in hot-spot areas; therefore, the cameras were perceived as ineffective by some staff as they did not capture violent acts occurring in hot-spot areas. Linked to this, staff had different ideas about what constituted hot-spot areas of the ward and therefore believed that cameras were needed in almost all areas of the ward, thereby increasing surveillance of patients inside it.

> S22: *"we've got the female lounge is covered. The male corridor is not! The airlock is covered by three different cameras. The office is not! We've got about nine cameras in various places outside that we don't need to look at erm the dining room is not! We have cameras in all the rooms in the ECA [Extra Care Area] we don't have cameras in these rooms off err side rooms. Very odd!"*

The expansion of CCTV cameras in site 2 was instigated following an incident in the communal area of the ward, where there was no CCTV coverage because it was not a blind-spot. However, it was a hot-spot area where patients were likely to get aggressive because there was more interaction with other patients or staff with whom they might disagree with. On this site, the rationale for additional cameras throughout the hot-spot areas of the ward was driven by an incident in the ward where a staff member was injured and blamed the hospital for their injury. The lack of cameras covering this area and the poor coverage provided by existing cameras became the impetus to expand camera surveillance into all parts of the ward, including those areas that were neither hot-spots nor blind-spots. The driver here for expanding camera surveillance was predicted on the potential of the cameras to capture incidents in as many parts of the ward as possible. Marx (1988) raises the question as to who benefits from this expansion. The expansion of cameras in this way also influences how risk is prioritised. By expanding camera function from blind-spots to hot-spots, the cameras also act as agents in protecting the hospital as an organisation. Chapter 4 examines how this influences nursing care inside the mental health ward.

Zero tolerance

Manager's concern about incidents of violence and aggressive behaviour from patients towards staff and sometimes other patients was a feature in all three sites. These incidents impact negatively not only on the patient who has lost control but also on staff and managers. Managers described how incidents of aggression and violence had led to the loss of time from work and, where staff had been seriously injured, to compensation claims. Although it is the case that in our everyday life we have a right not to be attacked (Macnish, 2014), the ward environment is different in that it has patients inside it who are angry, frustrated, have little control over their behaviour, feel they have nothing to lose and who therefore are more prone to becoming aggressive and possibly violent. This focus on aggression inside modern mental health hospitals has steadily gained momentum since 1999 when the Department of Health introduced a Health Service Circular in which they announced a campaign to stop violence against those staff working in the NHS. This policy was referred to as a campaign for zero tolerance of violence to NHS staff. The policy was aimed at stopping violence inside all hospitals, including mental health hospitals. Most managers generally agreed that while the notion of zero tolerance to violence continues to be promoted in general hospitals, this is not as easy to enforce in mental hospitals.

> M5: *"Zero tolerance policy within mental health is very difficult to manage for all sorts of different reasons. One's mental state doesn't necessarily allow people [patients] to understand the elements of the policy ... and equally there are times where other systems don't necessarily support the implication of zero tolerance. So the idea that the police would respond to an incident within and A@E [Accident and Emergency] structure, for instance, in a zero tolerance way is probably very different to dealing with somebody in a mental health unit, who's detained under the Mental Health Act, who's not deemed to have mental capacity. There are all sorts of issues around zero tolerance policies".*

In supporting staff and patients from aggressive patients, managers found themselves in positions where they were taking on simultaneously different, and at times, conflicting roles. For example, they were placed in positions where they were an investigator when incidents happened inside the ward, as someone who provided staff and possibly the patient with support at a distressing time, sometimes as the person involved in any disciplinary action or learning process and at other times the person involved in instigating criminal proceedings. This placed frontline managers in a difficult position when upholding the fundamental values of mental health nursing while resisting organisational response for more CCTV. In these situations, it is not difficult to see how prevailing discourses around risk management override the therapeutic benefits of mental health nursing.

> M9: *"... depending on when the next serious incident is, and what the characteristics of it are ... you know, there is a SI [serious incident] of some sort, erm people can't see exactly what happened. We had somebody that stumbled fell backwards and banged their head and had err erm bleed, and at that point that they'd fallen backwards they were being escorted into their room [bedroom]. This was about, I don't know, two years ago. Something like that, err and anyway there was plenty of witness evidence and I think he was okay in the end, and he himself said what had happened but the corridor wasn't covered. And initially, I mean the cynics and those ... you know, how do you know he wasn't pushed, tripped up, jumped upon, set upon, whatever. No CCTV, we ought to have it".*

M9's example suggests that policies and practices designed to protect patients and staff become hijacked by the organisation where protecting the reputation of the hospital takes precedence. The idea that casting the surveillance net wider inside the ward will protect patients and staff is a way of protecting the organisation. This agenda becomes ever increasingly important as inpatient mental health care moves further into private and independent hospital care where reputations matter because they come with financial risks. Therefore, the relevancy of zero tolerance policies as questioned by M5 continue to dominate where it is the belief that only those mental health wards where there is no violence are safe wards. In the meantime, as surveillance expands inside wards, what is classed as an incident or a serious incident also has the capacity to change and expand as more behaviours become less tolerated. Chapter 4 discusses in more detail how this can affect staff relationships with patients.

CCTV and patient justice

The negative link between some mental health conditions and technologies is quite common. Cruickshank (cited in Freeman and Freeman, 2008: 12) (below) describes his own experience of paranoia about technology:

> I believed everything and everyone were put in my path as some sort of psychological test. I believed I had mini cameras implanted in my eyes and that there was a control room somewhere with people analysing

> the data they saw through my eyes. I believed the crows around me were designed to follow me unobtrusively.

Most managers recognised that some patients might perceive the cameras negatively because of their mental health condition.

> M2: *"I think that some people [staff] worried that it would make you feel more paranoid ... so if people [patients] are already frightened that they're being watched why would you put in a camera ... that obviously would make people [patients] more distressed ... that was the biggest one really about making people [patients] feel err spied upon and it would fuel paranoia".*

Some staff also believed that because of their mental health condition, some patients were likely to experience paranoia whether there was CCTV in the ward or not and, therefore, it was a moot point whether the cameras increased patient paranoia or not. Despite reservations about camera use inside the ward, other benefits of cameras took precedence in the final decision to implement them. Below, M10 describes how the cameras can benefit patients by creating equality inside the ward.

> M10: *"... it's a two-way street, it gives protection to staff, protection to service users [patients], erm that way everybody is, you know, they know it's there and it's looking after them all; it's not just looking after staff. It's not at all discriminatory".*

The idea that patients also have access to social justice from CCTV is limited. This limitation is demonstrated in the mental capacity of the patient to understand the context in which they are being observed as well as having access to affordable legal support, and as patient P4 explains:

> P4: *"Misbehaviour by staff is not at the forefront. It is only patients who misbehave".*

Also inside all three sites, apart from their use inside bedrooms, patients were not told that there were CCTV cameras present in communal areas of the ward. Contrary to Data Protection Act (1998) and Information Commissioner's Office Code of Practice (2017), none of the three sites had signs inside the ward to inform patients, staff and visitors to the ward that the PICU used camera surveillance. Some managers believed that there should be CCTV signage inside the ward to warn patients, while other managers were surprised that the ward and the unit did not have signs. Several managers believed this should be remedied because it was contrary to data protection legislation, while other managers believed that so long as patients were aware that there were cameras in the ward, this was sufficient.

> M4: "*... if there is CCTV, it's more about explaining what it looks like to a new patient. So, these [cameras] are here. They're only in here they're not in your bedroom or if they are in your bedroom this is what it's used for, this is how it's monitored or not monitored, you know so we don't sit and watch you. But it is explained, we believe, whether this happens on a day-to-day basis, I don't know*".

The lack of documentation available to patients about the cameras, including how the cameras are used to maintain their safety, their right to not want to be monitored in this way or to complain about their use and how to access CCTV footage, places patients in an inequitable position. It was the taken-for-granted attitude adopted by some managers that the cameras were inside the ward for the benefit of patients and staff that resulted in the lack of information and choices given to them. While staff can walk away from the cameras at the end of their shift, patients have to remain in the ward until they are discharged. This makes the patient experience of cameras different to staff, managers and any visitors to the ward.

Conclusion

The trajectory of audits presented in this research suggests that more NHS hospitals are choosing to implement CCTV cameras inside mental health wards. The lack of national drivers for introducing CCTV cameras inside the ward has meant that decision-making has remained a local one. This chapter has identified several reasons for introducing cameras inside the ward. These include:

- Managing the reputation of the hospital and the Trust.
- Being ready for potential serious incidents which may or may not impact the Trust.
- As a knee-jerk response to an incident that has happened inside their hospital or another hospital.
- Managing political agendas around violence inside mental health wards.
- Safeguarding women patients inside mental health wards.
- Providing an alternative to night-time observation of patients.
- An expectation that because the unit is an intensive care facility that it should have cameras within it.

Most managers have treated CCTV cameras as a means of solving or managing ward concerns. Therefore, the negotiations between staff, patients and patient groups have centred on these concerns. The final chapter (Chapter 6) will gather together a further discussion of theory and practice.

Bibliography

Beck, U. (1992). *Risk Society: Towards a New Modernity*, London: Sage.

Care Quality Commission (CQC). (2018). *The Stare of Care in Mental Health Services 2014–2017: Findings from CQC's Programme of Comprehensive Inspections of Specialist Mental Health Services*, Care Quality Commission, Gallowgate, Newcastle-upon-Tyne, England.

Chambers, M. and Gillard, S. (2005). *Review of CCTV on John Meyer Ward, 19 July 2005 Agenda Item 9, South West London and St George's NHS Mental Health Trust*, South West London and St George's NHS Mental Health Trust Board Meeting, 28 July 2005, London.

Deluze, G. and Guattari, F. (1980). *A Thousand Plateaus*, translated by Brian Massumi, New York: University of Minnesota Press.

Department of Health (DH). (1999). *Campaign to Stop Violence against Staff Working in the NHS: NHS Zero Tolerance HSC 1999/226*, London: Department of Health.

Department of Health (DH). (2002). *Women's Mental Health: Into the Mainstream Strategic Development for Mental Health Care for Women*, London: Department of Health.

Department of Health (DH). (2013). *Health Building Note 03–01: Adult acute mental health units*. Available online: www.nationalarchives.gov.uk/doc/open-government-licence/ [accessed 10 February 2019].

Desai, S. (2009). "The new stars of CCTV: What is the purpose of monitoring patients in communal areas of psychiatric hospital wards, bedrooms and seclusion rooms?" *Diversity in Health and Care*, 6(1): 45–53.

Freeman, D. and Freeman, J. (2008). *Paranoia: The Twenty-First Century Fear*, Oxford: Oxford University Press.

Giddens, A. (1998). *The Third Way: The Renewal of Social Democracy*, Cambridge: Polity Press.

Gilligan, C. (1982). *In a Different Voice: Psychological Theory and Women's Development*, Cambridge: Harvard University Press.

Goffman, E. (1969). *The Presentation of the Self in Everyday Life,* Great Britain: Allen Lane, Penguin Press.

Information Commissioner's Office. (2017). *In the Picture: A Data Protection Code of Practice for Surveillance Cameras and Personal Information*, Wilmslow, Cheshire, England: Information Commissioner's Office.

Jørgensen, K. and Rendtorff, J.D. (2017). "Patient participation in mental health care – Perspectives of healthcare professionals: An integrated review," *Scandinavian Journal of Caring Sciences*, 31(2): 490–501.

Kelly, M.G.E. (2009). *The Political Philosophy of Michel Foucault*, Oxon: Routledge.

Koskela, H. (2012). "'You shouldn't wear that body': The problematic of surveillance and gender," in K. Ball, K.D. Haggerty and D. Lyon (eds), *Routledge Handbook of Surveillance Studies.* London: Routledge, pp. 49–56.

Laurance, J. (2005). "Health Trust is fined after a mentally ill patient kills a nurse," *The Independent*, 6 May 2005. Available online: www.independent.co.uk/life-style/health-and-families/health-news/health-trust-is-fined-after-mentally-ill-patient-kills-nurse-495266.html [accessed 17 September 2018].

Lyon, D. (1994). *The Electronic Eye: The Rise of Surveillance Society*, Minnesota: University of Minnesota Press.

Macnish, K. (2014). "Just surveillance: Towards a normative theory of surveillance," *Surveillance and Society*, 12(1): 142–153.

Marx, G.T. (1988). *Undercover: Police Surveillance in America*, Berkley: University of California.

Marx, G.T. (2001). "Murky conceptual waters: The public and the private," *Ethics and Information Technology*, 3: 157–169.

McCahill, M. (2012). "Crime, surveillance and media," in K. Ball, K.D. Haggerty, and D. Lyon (eds), *Routledge Handbook of Surveillance Studies*, London: Routledge, 244–250.

Monahan, T. (2011). "Surveillance as cultural practice," *The Sociological Quarterly*, 52(4): 495–508.

National Association of Psychiatric Intensive and Low Secure Care Units (NAPICU). (2014). *National Minimum Standards for Psychiatric Intensive Care in General Adult Services*, East Kilbride: NAPICU International Press.

National Association of Psychiatric Intensive and Low Secure Care Units (NAPICU). (2017). *Design Guidance for Psychiatric Intensive Care Units,* East Kilbride: NAPICU International Press.

Stolovy, T., Melamed, Y. and Afek, A. (2015). "Video surveillance in mental health facilities: Is it ethical?" *The Israel Medical Association Journal*, 17(5): 274–276.

Taylor, E. (2010). "I spy with my little eye: The use of CCTV in schools and the impact of privacy," *Sociological Review*, 58(3): 381–405.

Tully, J., Fahy, T. and Larkin, F. (2016). "New technologies in the management of risk and violence in forensic settings," in K.D. Warburton and S.M. Stahl, (eds), *Violence and Psychiatry*. Cambridge: Cambridge University Press, pp. 314–322.

Warr, J., Page, M. and Crossen-White, H. (2005). *The Appropriate Use of Closed Circuit Television (CCTV) in a Secure Unit*, Study undertaken by Montpellier Unit and Bournemouth University, England.

Webster, C.W.R. (2009). "CCTV policy in the UK: Reconsidering the evidence base," *Surveillance and Society*, 6(1): 10–22.

Chapter 4

Practice implications and CCTV surveillance

Introduction

To understand how CCTV as a technological tool is used inside the ward, it is not sufficient to just examine what it does but also how human beings give meaning to its function. McCahill and Norris (2003: 46) have referred to this as the "human mediation of technology". Verbeek (2016: 190) claims that technologies are not "merely functional and instrumental objects", rather they are "mediators of human experiences and practices". He goes on to suggest that to gain a full understanding of a technological tool, including CCTV, it is important to examine how human beings give meaning to these mediations. To do this, he suggests that it is important to examine technology both empirically and conceptually.

This chapter includes the uses of CCTV which have been endorsed by the National Association of Psychiatric Care and Low Secure Units (or NAPICU) and those uses of cameras that have evolved inside the ward as a result of them being available to staff. The cameras were generally welcomed by staff in all three research sites as they aided them with a range of activities inside the ward including carrying out nursing observations more efficiently, keeping an eye on peers, carrying out unobtrusive observations and so on. This chapter examines not only a range of these practices but also how camera use has influenced staff relationships with patients, peers and managers.

Background

NAPICU's guidance is one of the very few documents that suggest how CCTV technology can be used inside the mental health ward. The guidance is endorsed by NAPICU as a professional body, who, according to their website, is a registered charity established in 1996 and whose primary interest is the development and improvement of PICUs and low secure services. One of their aims is to provide best practice guidance in association with a range of national bodies. The document, "*National Minimum Standards for Psychiatric Intensive Care in General Adult Services*", referred to within this

DOI: 10.4324/9781003179306-4

chapter, has been endorsed by several professional bodies, including the Royal College of Psychiatrists and the Royal College of Nurses (NAPICU, 2014). This guidance is not embedded in any one piece of legislation but is informed by a range of legislation, including the Data Protection Act 1998. The document cites the following recommendations on the use of CCTV:

> *7.2.74. Units should consider the potential value of CCTV as an area of innovation within a PICU in certain circumstances and areas in which it could be carefully deployed.*
>
> *7.2.75. CCTV has proved useful by providing the following:*
>
> - *Additional options for observation in difficult to supervise areas (e.g. gardens, smoking areas);*
> - *A means of evidence, recording untoward incidents, potential offences or investigating allegations;*
> - *An additional means by which staff can review the management of difficult situations;*
> - *Up-to-date pictures of patients who may have absconded and are considered at risk.*
>
> *7.2.76. The CCTV recording system should be easily accessible by designated staff with the appropriate training.*
>
> *7.2.77. Any use of CCTV should be compliant with all data protection and other CCTV related legislation.*
>
> (Quoted from NAPICU, 2014: 30)

The same document also recommends the use of infrared CCTV camera technology and audio equipment inside patient bedrooms:

> *7.2.70. There are products available that allow alternative methods of regular night time observation with the aim of minimising disturbance and maximising privacy (e.g. infrared, breathing monitors). The value of such products should be considered in diminishing the disturbance caused by regular interval (usually a minimum of hourly) night time observation.*
>
> (Quoted from NAPICU, 2014: 29)

A further document, NAPICU and NHS Clinical Commissioners (2016: 13) also suggests that CCTV should be considered as an observation tool to supervise (section 17) leave authorised by a patient's responsible clinician for those patients detained under mental health legislation around the hospital periphery:

> *3.31. To facilitate safe access to outside areas for patients including those on Section 17 leave, a number of safeguards are needed:*

- *Consideration of appropriate staff supervision, engagement and other observation (including use of CCTV) given the mix and number of patients outside or on leave at any one time.*

There are two interesting points to consider about this guidance. First, by suggesting that PICUs should consider CCTV as "an area of innovation", NAPICU has built into its guidance the notion of function creep in that it invites NHS Trusts to seek out further uses for the technology (2014: 7.2.74). Second, as these innovative uses of CCTV become established practice, they become part of future guidance endorsing its uses. For example, the use of cameras in hospital grounds to monitor section 17 (or authorised) leave is now approved in the document NHS Clinical Commissioners guidance (2016), where CCTV use is presented as a desirable tool in the monitoring of leave immediately outside hospital grounds.

Surveillance creep

Bijker (1995) claims that the expansion of CCTV and changes in its function happen because its uses are interpretive and therefore not confined by imagination or creativity. He suggests this is because information systems (CCTV) together with their information content can be used in multiple ways. The term function creep was coined by Winner (1977) to describe how technology intended for one purpose is used for a different one. Marx (1988) coined the term surveillance creep while researching his book "*Undercover: Police Surveillance in America*". Similar to Winner's function creep, Marx used the term surveillance creep to denote the use of technology ascribed for one purpose being used for another. However, Marx specifically makes a distinction between the uses of surveillance technologies as a means of expanding surveillance through surveillance creep, whereas Winner's (1977) notion of function creep is not necessarily tied to this.

Haggerty (2012: 236) describes the dynamics of surveillance creep in the context of the police force where aspects such as snitching are described as "low-tech" surveillance and use of CCTV cameras as "high-tech" surveillance. He provides an example of how local authorities have used high-tech surveillance technology (CCTV), which was initially authorised to counter terrorism, to regulate low-level crimes, such as "people putting their garbage out on the wrong day, not cleaning up after their dog, urinating in public...", and thereby increasing everyday surveillance practices (Haggerty, 2012: 241). Dahl and Sætnan (2009: 88) claim that function creep happens because surveillance techniques are open to interpretation and thereby open to new areas of use and that once CCTV is in place, it seems wasteful not to use it to its "fullest acceptable limit". It is this, they claim, which leads to a shift in the "moral terrain" once a new function has been introduced. These views linked to CCTV surveillance suggest two main concerns of CCTV use. First, the notion of function creep suggests that the interpretative nature of the cameras means that their uses are wider than what they were originally designed to achieve or, in the case of the research sites, what managers may have initially wanted them to achieve. Second, all functional uses of cameras can change relationships inside the ward. This includes staff relationships with patients, with one another and managers.

CCTV and difficult-to-observe areas

Exposing blind-spots

According to the Collins English Dictionary (1979),

> A blind-spot is an area in your range of vision that you cannot see properly but which you really should be able to see. For example, when you are driving a car, the area just behind your shoulders is often a blind-spot.

The phrase blind-spot was used figuratively by managers and staff as a shorthand way to describe difficult-to-supervise areas inside the ward. These areas included corridors or spaces where it was not possible to maintain a visual eye on the patient at all times usually because of structural constraint. In his research inside asylums, Goffman (1961: 204) described some spaces inside the ward which he believed were "ruled by less than usual staff authority", and it is these areas that would have been classed as blind-spots because they were not always easy to physically supervise. Blind-spot areas are associated with the architectural design of buildings, and often older buildings are thought to have more areas within them that are difficult to supervise. For example, inside one research site, it was not possible to see the whole garden area from the ward office as this area extended around a corner. This led to patients conducting activities in that area that they may not have in supervised areas.

> Field note 018: "*Patient (white, male) enters garden area. He walks past me, goes to the side/back of garden and urinates against a wall. Walks past me again – doesn't say anything … Speak to staff x about this – why no CCTV there – she says it is a blind-spot and management know about this but don't do anything*".

While NAPICU (2014) guidance sanctions the use of CCTV to open up difficult-to-supervise areas, what is classed as a difficult-to-supervise area or a blind-spot was a point of disagreement between managers and staff (as raised in Chapter 3). For example, some managers believed that CCTV cameras should not be used in those areas of the ward where staff should be physically present, or supervised areas, and in those areas where staff have clear sightlines:

> M5: *"Cos as I said it's not used predominantly for observation. It shouldn't be used for observation".*

However, in their desire to maintain a constant vigilant eye on patients, what constituted a blind-spot differed for staff who believed that any area which could not be seen at all times constituted a blind-spot. In these instances, staff were not always concerned about how the cameras might affect patients. They were more concerned about maintaining visual contact with each patient so that they had an overview of where each patient was located in the context of the ward.

> S7: *"I think they are a benefit because you can't have eyes in the back of your head, and the ward is so big. You need to have these cameras to be able to give you visual access to the different areas".*

Expanding blind-spot areas

In one research site, the dining room area was not covered by CCTV, which staff claimed was a blind-spot. However, managers believed that this area should be supervised by staff when patients are using it. It was often this disagreement between staff and managers which prompted some staff to change the status of certain spaces inside the ward that they believed were hot-spots for violence, to blind-spots. This was so that they could justify cameras within these areas. These staff, for example, believed that some patients knew that there were cameras inside the ward and deliberately targeted those areas where there were no cameras to become angry or aggressive, resulting in the displacement of aggression and violent behaviour away from CCTV cameras.

> S22: *"We have so many blind spots that just as many assaults happen off camera! So, it's not always massively err massively helpful in that respect".*
>
> S9: *"I do believe some of the patient's know that there's areas, that there are blind spots they probably don't know all the blind spots, but they've tried moving to different areas and getting angry".*
>
> S15: *"We tend to escort patients to their bedrooms umm but as soon as we're in those areas, we're out of sight of the cameras and things, and they tend to be where quite a lot of incidents can happen".*

The expansion of CCTV surveillance to include cameras in more areas of the ward raises some concerns. First, blind-spots are no longer linked to opening up difficult-to-supervise spaces. They become any space inside the ward where there are no cameras, and this further changes the nature of surveillance inside the ward. For example, staff can reduce face-to-face contact with patients as the cameras increasingly become how they observe patients. Second, having more cameras inside the ward can also influence how staff interact with patients and therefore change the nature of any therapeutic contact. Chapter 2 has highlighted existing studies (Chambers and Gillard, 2005; Warr et al., 2005) and how the cameras affect staff relationship with patients. For example, Chambers and Gillard's (2005) explanation of how some staff became reluctant to use therapeutic touch with patients in case this was misconstrued by other people looking at the CCTV monitor or CCTV footage. Below, S11 explains how she currently communicates with patients and how the addition of more cameras inside the ward might force her to change how she does this. This is because she feared how other staff and managers might interpret her communication with patients.

> S11: *"I try to make em laugh as much as I can or and sometimes it can verge, it can verge on a bit, do you know what I mean? On a bit, I don't know where, where one of the patients says shut up x [says own name] you're getting on my nerves and I say it back to em you shut up as well, but it's jest, it's joking, where if we had cameras like that it may be, it would pick up and not everybody would see that as, and then that's when it becomes, that's when my nursing will have to change then".*

In addition, the expansion of cameras also influences how staff tolerate and manage any violence and aggression inside the ward. The loss of temper by a patient is not located to environmental factors, for instance, the frustration of being locked up inside a ward, or living inside restricted and tight ward spaces. These behaviours are perceived as wilful acts by patients where the cameras are seen as an ally in consolidating an already existing narrative about the violent nature of patients who enter PICUs (Saverimuttu, 2000; Bowers et al., 2008; Bennett et al., 2011). Below, S22 describes the reason why she believes patients entering PICUs are different.

> S22: *"We're seeing cuts in other services and stuff like that a lot more. The people [patients] that we're working with here are no longer kind of strictly PICU patients, we're working with a lot more people [patients] that are actually erm people that have fallen through the cracks where there are no services specific to them anymore. So, the client groups changed a bit ..."*

In this way, the cameras also became a means of proving to managers and others that the needs of mental health patients had changed. For some staff, these patients with dependency on alcohol and substance misuse were not strictly mental health patients. These staff believed that the PICU ward environment was not suitable for such patients who, they believed, required a different response.

CCTV and potential offences and allegations

CCTV and "true view"

Some frontline managers (see Chapter 3) believed that camera evidence should not be central to evidence gathering when an allegation has been made about a patient or a member of staff. However, when staff were required to provide verbal accounts and/or written accounts of what happened during a violent incident, several tended to believe that CCTV evidence was more reliable than written and verbal accounts. This was based on their belief that written and verbal accounts were open to interpretation, whereas camera footage would show what actually happened.

> S16: "*I would say I wouldn't feel safe, as daft as it sounds, I wouldn't feel safe, if, because personally uh if there was an incident and my err ability came into question. Err I would feel more confident in saying well you can check back and see that I did things right. So, you can see dah, dah, dah. If there was any question of my practice shall we say erm, so yeah, for that reason I'd like to think that they've done more good then they have bad*".

When a situation inside the ward became a wider concern, for example, when a patient became violent or aggressive, it was managers and not the consultant psychiatrist who dealt with these incidents. This sometimes created an anomaly for staff whose natural alliance when caring for patients is with the psychiatrist. Within the pastoral relationship, staff take their lead in how to effectively manage the care of each patient from the psychiatrist and not necessarily managers, especially those managers who are not frontline nursing staff. This anomaly is represented in the relationship between staff and managers. Whereas the psychiatrist might be more interested in knowing why the patient became aggressive, managers were more interested in how they, as staff, allowed the patient to become aggressive, and how they managed the situation. Hence, staff were often concerned about how managers would perceive their behaviour when an incident happened inside the ward. Also, as people who were responsible for their employment status in that managers could terminate their employment, they sometimes saw managers as a potential threat. Therefore, even though the cameras placed them under more surveillance, staff saw them as an ally in exonerating them. So much so, that any capture of a situation resulted in staff perceiving this as a "true view" of the circumstances (Cameron, 2004).

> S22: "*I have had erm CCTV used as part of an investigation … the CCTV was reviewed by the x Board of me searching the patient coming in cos they wanted to review whether I'd searched him erm in line with protocol, which I had … so yeah it was reviewed erm to sort of erm critique my practice,*

which luckily I did it right, and so, I've been on that end of it as well, where they are using it to try and see whether I've, I've acted wrongly".

According to Hope (2009), this suspicion facilitates target hardening where security measures become prioritised and any problems inside the ward that are linked to patient care are dealt with via system integration (or reliance on CCTV evidence), as opposed to social integration (or talking things out). As a result, the focus shifts from relationship building between staff and patients, and staff and managers, to reliance on CCTV, "to deter deviancy or facilitate punishment" (Hope, 2009: 902). Hope cites Garland (2001) to make the point that the implication of this is a shift in values where "crime and deviancy become perceived as mundane, inevitable everyday occurrences", where the organisation begins to categorise patients and staff in the context of the risk they pose (Hope, 2009: 903). As staff felt more under suspicion, it also affected how they perceived patients. It was the patient's negative behaviour that became the target for surveillance over behaviour that promoted their well-being.

S24: "*The one in the garden, a patient ... again its allegations. He threw himself onto the hedge ... for some reason he decided that he would just, he launched himself ... he made an allegation that a member of staff, he pushed me, and on the cameras, the staff member is on the other side of the garden and he just threw himself*".

Patient aggression as a crime

In his analysis of governmentality, Foucault (2009) believed that good government of subjects should not be reliant on the use of sovereign power (see Chapter 2). Therefore, staff inside the ward were always on the lookout for any potentially volatile situations. This was so that they could intervene before the situation got out of control, and they had to then rely on the use of seclusion, or other interventions, such as use of additional medication or full-body restraint. Therefore, staff expected violence inside these wards and were on the lookout for any violent situations erupting. They did this so that they could intervene quickly to manage any problems before things got out of hand.

S6: *"cos it's just a more secure environment. Hmm we've got more risky patients so I guess they [meaning managers] think a lot more things can go wrong here than acute wards".*

S18: *"because of the risk here because there is a high risk of violence, obviously that's part of the criteria, part of the criteria for this place".*

The idea that the type of patient that was being cared for inside the PICU was more "risky" and prone to aggression meant that most staff expected the ward to have cameras. The availability of CCTV footage as evidence also influenced staff expectations as to how the criminal justice system should respond to violent situations. For example, during fieldwork observations inside one site, police were contacted on three occasions to remove a male patient from the ward because he had assaulted other patients and staff. This patient was taken to the local police station and returned to the ward often on the same day, or the following day. On one occasion, his assaultive behaviour was partly captured on CCTV footage, and staff were annoyed when police decided not to prosecute the patient and instead returned him to the ward. Managers in this situation were not so concerned about whether the police prosecuted the patient or not. They were more concerned about reporting the incident to the correct authority. However, using CCTV as an additional form of evidence gathering prompted staff to view any act of violence and aggression with less tolerance. This led some staff to believe that all acts of violence by patients were done knowingly. Therefore, these staff disregarded other reasons such as a patient feeling frustrated with their environment, or because a patient might be upset with a particular staff member, or because the patient was denied access to their belonging, or because the aggression was associated with their mental health condition as potential reasons for the patient becoming aggressive.

> S22: "*We've had a number of incidents where we've had patients, who have capacity with regards to violent behaviour erm committing assaults against staff members. We've then submitted the CCTV along with statements to the police and still gets dropped for lack of evidence*".

The reporting of violent attacks to the police also meant that violence became a prominent issue inside the ward. Below, a staff member describes how the hospital deals with incidents of violence by encouraging the reporting of it to the police.

> S14: "*It [CCTV] does help in that respect and again I suppose it benefits the patients because if they're being hurt then, and they want to press charges with the police, which we do encourage that on here, if they're, if they're assaulted by another patient*".

Gilburt et al. (2008: 4) describe a range of ways in which patients experience frustration inside mental health wards. In their research, patients attributed coercive activities inside the ward as points of their frustration. This included being detained under mental health legislation where they did not see detention as a legal process but instead as a coercive event. Coercion also included the tension between having to behave in a certain way, referred to by patients as "playing the game", and the use of non-physical force, for example, being coerced into taking medication. It is these subtle and not so subtle coercive practices inside the ward that patients found frustrating. Field notes from ethnographic observations for this research identified a range of situations inside the ward where patients were left in powerless positions, for example, when staff made arrangements with patients for authorised (section 17) leave arrangements, where this leave off the ward can only happen if the patient is accompanied by staff, was cancelled at the last minute. Although the staff themselves may also be powerless in these situations often because leave would be cancelled as a result of the ward being short-staffed, patients, who were desperate to have time away from the ward, did not always empathise with their reasons. Some staff found it difficult when patients did not empathise with them, and they did not always appreciate that having leave off the ward was not just about getting away from the ward environment but also proving to others that they were ready for discharge. In this way, staff did not always understand the importance for patients to prove their readiness to be discharged from the ward.

Quirk et al. (2006) highlight the permeability of the modern mental health ward environment where they say relationships are not fixed and are transitory. For example, PICUs as intensive care units were designed to provide intensive support to patients for a short period. Therefore, some patients spent as little as one week in the ward and others up to three to four months or even longer after which they were discharged into the community, moved to an acute ward or moved to a secure care facility. How long each patient would spend inside a PICU was vague as it was not easy to predict recovery. The unpredictability of not knowing how long they would be inside the ward impacted how patients and staff committed to getting to know one another. Also, the nature of shift patterns where the core nursing team changed every shift was equally problematic in forming relationships. Inside all three research sites, shift patterns changed three times, with a morning shift, afternoon shift and night shift. During fieldwork observations, despite being inside each ward at different times of each day and night throughout an eight- to ten-week period, there were staff whom, after an initial meeting with them, I never saw again. The fluidity of the staff in this way meant that it was difficult for staff and patients to form any attachments and most shifts, especially in those wards which relied heavily on bank and agency staff; it also meant that patients were often cared for by people who did not know them. The outcome of this constant turnover of staff inside all three wards meant that it was difficult for patients to form relationships with staff and vice versa.

The transitory nature of nursing care also produced conflicting practices resulting in additional stresses for staff, who are placed in a position in which any action that they take is perceived as unsatisfactory by the organisation. It also creates a burden on staff who are placed in a situation where their role as caregivers becomes undermined by their role as potential informants. During any incidence in the ward where a patient has lost control, staff are expected to record the patient presentation and their mental health, what circumstances led to the encounter, how the patient became irritable, how they became aggressive, what damage they caused inside the ward and so on. This reporting of the behaviours of patients also gradually influences therapeutic relationships. This is because constantly documenting a patient's behaviour, rather than attempting to understand why a patient might inappropriately respond under pressure, results in a discrete mind shift each time where the patient is no longer perceived as a vulnerable individual but is instead seen as someone who is a danger and security risk inside the ward.

This subtle dual role places staff in an uneasy situation, where they are not only responsible for patient care, but they are also increasingly made more responsible for maintaining security inside the ward. Ball et al. (2015: 51) believe that this is a result of the de-politicisation of security, which they suggest result in security measures becoming "diffused into everyday life". The diffusion of security measures inside the ward was evident in staff responsibility for patient behaviours and actions. As these security measures begin to influence practices inside the ward, some staff begin to have less empathy with certain patient behaviours, where they believe that any aggressive encounters should be reported to the police because they threaten the ward environment. For these staff, CCTV evidence took on greater significance. The diffusion of security measures inside the ward also benefitted managers as staff recognised how seriously managers took the reporting of incidents inside it. Below, S18, who has had no experience of being involved in an incident where CCTV evidence has been used, describes how CCTV evidence was treated in another case. This process has an added advantage in that staff are also reminded that they too are under surveillance.

> S18: *"I haven't seen it properly, the process go through, but I've seen the CDs where it says like evidence for, and, you know, it's marked CCTV cameras ... I haven't done the process but I've seen the CD in a case that is evidence for a case that's happening or going through".*

CCTV and difficult situations

Constructing a narrative

NAPICU (2014) guidance suggests that CCTV can aid in the understanding of an event or incident inside the ward. This is so that staff can learn from any incidents and reduce or eliminate any potential triggers or threats from the ward. NHS England requires Mental Health Trusts to record untoward incidents and serious untoward incidents inside wards as part of a wider drive to reduce risk factors that undermine safety. They define a serious untoward incident as:

> events in health care where the potential for learning is so great, or the consequences to patients, families and carers, staff or organisations are

> so significant, that they warrant using additional resources to mount a comprehensive response. Serious incidents can extend beyond incidents which affect patients directly and include incidents which may indirectly impact patient safety or an organisation's ability to deliver ongoing healthcare.
>
> (NHS England, 2010: 12)

Staff provided several examples that they identified as serious untoward incidents inside the ward.

> S9: "*Basically a patient, a male patient, actually attempted to strangle another patient and luckily thank goodness, it was in front of the camera and we were able to, we were able to timeline it, and show exactly what actually occurred prior to that event happening, and what happened after the event*".
>
> S16: "*I've seen it plain as day, like one [patient] was out the, erm the activity room. For example, err this inner door was kicked, then the wrought-back outer door was kicked, a chair was quickly brought out the back and then despite it being, I should imagine incredibly difficult, this person [patient] had still managed to shimmy up over the top and was gone. And you could see it, plain as the day, and it didn't seem to matter a jot that there was a camera watching them all the time*".

If it was available, staff tended to use CCTV to construct a narrative when there was an incident in the ward that involved them.

> S8: "*When it came down to the paperwork, we had to pause it, look who was where, on what arm, at what time, and during the restraint … cos so many members of [staff] no one could possibly remember that!*"
>
> S15: "*So the movements [of the patient] were monitored previous the incident, and then the build-up just before it erm, to try and find out where he got the cord from. If he had to go looking for it, that kind of thing*".

Creating a safe ward environment

Staff also used CCTV footage to learn from incidents including sometimes how they could and should have responded differently. This learning was not only about their responses, but it was also about how to make the ward a more secure place so that patients inside it could be kept safe. In the examples below, without CCTV footage, staff would not have the same opportunity to learn best practice in the carrying out of restraint or find out how a patient managed to abscond from the ward so that it could not easily happen again. In the final example, staff would not have known that a patient had attempted to strangle another patient because in that situation it was a third patient who had intervened to stop the attack. Therefore, for some staff, the desire to learn from an incident was linked to securing the ward environment to provide safer care for all patients inside it.

> S8: "*We sort of like had a de-brief afterwards, um you know, you look at where everybody was. You sort of reflect on what happened and things, which I always find is good closure because it can be distressing, not just for the patients but for staff as well. It really can be!*".
>
> S11: "*We had a patient absconded the one night … and we couldn't think where they got out from, so we, of course, we're gonna, we're gonna, you know … myself and the nurse-in-charge went in there [ward managers office] to rewind it, to have a look to see where they got out …*".
>
> S11: "*… like two years ago we had a young male [patient] actually trying to strangle a female [patient] with erm, with erm piece of clothing, which was made up like a rope really … that he literally put round her neck … he was strangling her…and there was this other patient … did step in and stopped it …*".

Understanding patient behaviour

The need to secure the environment to make it a safer place for all patients was also linked to understanding patient behaviour better. In one research site, it was the role of a staff member to review minor incidents inside the ward. This staff described how she sometimes used CCTV footage as a learning tool to assess triggers for each patient who was involved in any altercation or restraint inside the ward. This was so that other staff could learn how to better interact with that patient, thereby avoiding the need for more coercive intervention such as seclusion, time out in an extra-care area, full-body restraint or forced medication. While managers might have perceived this as a reduction of risk factors inside the ward, staff wanted to understand the stressors for each patient and their reactions to events and triggers so that they could better interact with them. For staff, this intervention was more akin to their therapeutic role in nursing patients. Most staff welcomed this intervention as this understanding meant that they also did not have to take an aggressive stance with certain patients while they were involved in day-to-day interactions with them. Therefore, the cameras fulfil the potential for security and provide staff with a means of interacting more productively with patients.

> S22: "*So I will go back through and have a look at incidents where restraints have happened, and have a look and see like, has everything been done as it should have been, and sort of do a little bit of reflection and use it for debriefing and things like that … so I'll go back and look over incidents, and go like aw okay so that looked a little bit hairy, maybe next time we can try*

and maybe go into a different area, or we can try and step, sort of help, you go back a little bit further and you can look for any early warning signs and things like that".

CCTV and night-time observation

Using cameras inside bedrooms

Research site 3 decided to place an infrared CCTV camera and audio equipment inside each patient bedroom. These bedroom cameras were commonly referred to as an "INOP" system by staff, which was short hand for infrared night-time observation panel. The cameras did not record and could only be accessed by staff who used a fob key to operationalise them during their routine nursing observation of each patient during the night. Each time the camera is operational, a red light turns on inside the patient's bedroom. This alerts the patient that the camera is operational. The camera is located behind a small viewing box placed inside the bedroom wall and is configured to primarily view the patient's bed. Staff cannot move the angle of the camera, for example, to see other areas of the bedroom such as the en-suite bathroom or zoom in and out. It was also possible to hear the patient breathing when the audio equipment was switched on separately. The audio equipment was not connected to the camera. The CCTV monitor and audio equipment were located outside each patient bedroom door inside a box mounted on the wall. The staff could switch the cameras and audio equipment on as many times as they liked as the operationalisation of the cameras was not audited anywhere. Staff were therefore required to manually document that they had undertaken an observation of each patient when doing nurse observations.

Unless specified, all patients were routinely observed throughout the night at hourly intervals. Some staff believed that checking patients inside their bedroom using CCTV was a safer way of undertaking these routine night-time observations. This was mainly because there were patients who became angry and annoyed when the staff switched on the light and entered their room every hour. As a result, the cameras had a double advantage in that they allowed patients to gain a good night's sleep and kept staff safe while they were doing their job of monitoring patients. Therefore, the beneficial aspects of bedroom cameras were not only extended to patients, but also the staff.

> S21: "*some people [patients] can get agitated by it [night-time observations]. If you've got, if they're on like high observations, like every 15 minutes it's kind of, obviously be quite annoying if someone like keeps knocking your door, coming into your room every 15 minutes*".
>
> S22: "*it is [night-time observations] a source of conflict and it certainly was on the acute wards erm when back then they didn't even have observation windows so you would have to open a patient's door, turn the light on and turn it off, and that was really disruptive*".

Doubting the cameras

Despite the perceived benefits to themselves and patients of doing night-time observations using bedroom cameras, there were still staff who doubted what they were watching on CCTV monitors. These staff sometimes took an over cautionary approach to their observations using both the INOP system and manually checking, by switching the light on and/or opening the bedroom door, or the louvered observation panel located on the bedroom door. Some staff did this because they feared that their professionalism would come into question if a patient died during the night when they were involved in monitoring them. This fear negated the benefits of the cameras.

> S21: "*I mean if you're unsure you can always check the camera and if you feel like uncertain, you can always knock the door and say like you okay, like have a look in, or even do the window [observation panel] instead*".
>
> S23: "*I will look through the thing [observation panel] and I will put the lights on because obviously, it's our work, isn't it? And if I'm not sure, yeah ... last year I found a girl who committed suicide on my ward ... I think experiencing that, finding someone and going through the process writing statements, investigations, and coroner's court. It made me I think even more vigilant making sure I see someone properly, yeah*".
>
> S26: "*If there's ... someone's say suicidal for instance and you couldn't really see them with their blankets and everything I wouldn't just use that [INOP system]. I'd use that and I'd go in if I felt that I had to, if I couldn't see enough on the camera before I go in*".

Koskela (2000: 250) suggests that staff who are watching behind the cameras also find them equally disorientating and alienating. This is because she believes that the "alienated who look from behind the camera see the space under surveillance through the monitor (simplified to two dimensions) and they look at people as if they were objects". For some staff, this two-dimensional watching did not sit easily with their brief of maintaining a watchful eye on the patient throughout the night. For these staff, looking at the patient through the lens of a camera did not constitute a caring therapeutic gaze and was instead a look that was reduced to their bodily movements. This caused them some unease, and they did not feel they could trust what they were watching especially where a patient breathed inaudibly, and where there was little movement from them while they were sleeping. In these situations, staff did not always feel that the cameras were an enabling tool in monitoring patients.

However, by entering the patient's bedroom, they were also diminishing what the managers saw as the positive benefits of the system, which was for patients to get a good night's sleep without disturbance. Also, whether a patient had agreed to be observed in this way or not, staff carried out night-time observations in ways that they believed was most appropriate. For example, patient consent was required to use the infrared camera and audio equipment. Where consent was given, the phrase "INOP" would be written on a whiteboard mounted outside each patient bedroom door. This would indicate to any staff undertaking night-time observations that the patient had consented to be observed via infrared CCTV. Where this was not the case, the words "trad", short for traditional observations, would be noted on the white-board. Staff members that were observed as part of fieldwork observations inside the ward generally used their judgement as to how they did night-time nursing observations.

> Field note 223: "*Went around the ward with staff x doing traditional and INOP observations. There are 7 patients on the ward but only 1 patient has agreed to INOP. Staff x tells me that he sometimes uses INOP system even if a patient has asked for traditional obs. He says he does this when he knows the patient is asleep. He does this because he does not want to disturb the patient by switching on their bedroom light. I watch staff x use INOP system to carry out obs [observations] on 3 patients in addition to the one that has agreed to INOP. One of the patients is awake and sitting on a chair watching tv ... Staff x tells me that he knows that this patient is okay about staff using INOP because he has spoken to him*".

The efficacy of bedroom cameras was therefore undermined by staff's fear that they could be blamed if a patient died during the night while they were on duty.

Overriding consent

By choosing to do night-time observations in ways which they believed was appropriate for them meant that staff undermined patient's right to be observed in their bedroom in the way that they had consented. This annoyed some patients who were aware that staff did this.

> P11: "*They can be switched on or off ... and they tend to switch them on or off (laughs) regardless of what you say ... Intrusive really ... This environment ... you have the cameras, you also have the windows with people [staff] looking through, at times it's like being in prison. You're being inspected all the time. It's not very good*".
>
> P12: "*now I've noticed you can see a red light that comes on when they're using it and they rarely use it cos they can see you through the shutter [observation panel] anyway. They turn the light on at night ... they'll open the shutter and if the lights turned off they turn the light on and off again just to see you, which is like, you've got your camera, use the camera. Like, don't turn the light on when I'm sleeping!*"

For some patients, not knowing exactly how staff were observing them while they were inside their bedroom created stress. For these patients, the anticipatory conformity of the cameras was apparent in their belief that they were being watched constantly by bedroom cameras even during the day (Norris and Armstrong, 1999).

> P12: "*When I first came here it was a week or so until someone actually told me that they don't look at the CCTV in my room … and so, what for the first two weeks I was under the impression that I was being watched and they can just look at, check-in through, look in through, I thought they were watching in the office err so you know they could have explained that!*"

Gendered nature of camera use

Although managers provided a rationale for camera placement in female ward areas (see Chapter 3), there was less debate around the gendered nature of CCTV use inside bedrooms. It was the case in all three wards that both male and female staff did night-time observations of all patients regardless of their gender. Below, S27, a male member of staff, describes how uneasy he feels when observing female patients through the INOP system:

> S27: "*No one [patients] likes them [INOP cameras]. I don't think so, they don't. Yeah, even myself I wouldn't like it … it's particularly when we are doing the monitoring for the women. It becomes very … most of them will be their legs are out, open, erm the blankets fall off their body … when you check you just see her the way she is and that is not dignity really*".

This form of watching also has the potential to invoke feelings of loss of power associated with abuse that are often common with women's mental health. Karban (2011: 119) states that women's mental health is "more likely to be affected by the experience of violence and abuse, with a recognised association between domestic violence, depression, post-traumatic stress and self-harm". Koskela (2012: 52) suggests that CCTV surveillance can also turn the female body "into a sexualised object *without a mutual commitment* to such sexualisation". Therefore, women patients in these situations where they have no idea as to who is looking at them have to rely on the trust of the staff not to turn the watchful gaze into an abusive sexualised one. The fact that the INOP cameras do not record makes this additionally difficult to prove as there is no mechanism by which an independent person can tell how long a member of staff spent looking at a particular patient and why. The cameras in the communal female ward area did provide sightlines to female patient's bedroom doors; however, it was not possible to see staff using all INOP cameras, which were located next to each bedroom. Even where it was possible to view a staff member doing nurse monitoring using the INOP system in the female ward area, staff could easily justify their lingering gaze as necessary because it was not always easy to see the patient. However, while there was some monitoring of staff doing night-time observations in the female ward area, this was not the case in the male ward area where there was no camera coverage to capture staff using the INOP system.

CCTV and seclusion monitoring

The embarrassment of face-to-face looking

Several staff chose to use the camera in the seclusion room to monitor the patient in seclusion rather than doing face-to-face observations. These staff gave several reasons for this. Sometimes this was because there was not much happening, especially when the patient was either asleep and it was clear that they were sleeping, or because the patient was just sitting silently and doing little else. However, some staff believed that seclusion monitoring was more emotive than doing routine monitoring or observations inside the ward. These staff focused on the intensity of looking at the patient in seclusion and the discomfort of sitting in front of an almost full-length window panel, looking into the seclusion room. Below, S6 and S1 describe how uncomfortable they feel when they are sitting in front of the window panel and watching a patient inside the seclusion room. Unlike ward monitoring of patients where observation might mean a cursory glance at a patient every hour or half-hour, they believed that looking at the patient in seclusion was disrespectful because of the frequency of the look. In seclusion, staff were required to monitor the patient every five minutes. These staff frequently used the phrase "*it's rude to stare*" when talking about doing seclusion monitoring. The cameras, therefore, provided relief from this frequent watching of patients whom they believed also appreciated it. This is because as one staff described it, patients "*don't like to be stared at*". CCTV in this context took away the awkwardness out of having to do seclusion monitoring.

> S6: "*I guess people see CCTV as intrusive, I guess we, I sometimes find it less intrusive in the [de-escalation] room and seclusion room because rather than having to stare at them directly through a window and they know you're watching and they might feel uncomfortable, you can just kinda keep an eye on them on the screen. Sometimes I do feel like it's, don't know if they feel like it, but I definitely feel like it's less intrusive for me like having to stare at them through the window, whereas I can just keep an eye on them on CCTV*".
>
> S1: "*And then in the seclusion ... it's quite good cos sometimes your presence umm makes it worse actually for the patient. So you could use, sometimes it's like, there's a blind you can draw it and still watch them but you're not kind of staring through a window at them all the time, which I think, you know, some of them it helps*".

The watching of a patient was intensified in seclusion where the patient is seen not only by the camera but also by a staff member. Staff desire to not be rude, manage their awkwardness and genuinely attempting to give patients in seclusion some privacy meant that they tended to rely on the CCTV monitor to observe the patient. Some staff also preferred to close the blind in the window panel between the seclusion room and lobby or slightly sit away from the window panel so that the patient could not see them. This distanciation from the patient to manage the awkwardness of face-to-face looking also, at times, resulted in rude behaviour towards patients in seclusion by staff. For instance, it was ward policy that a member of staff would observe the patient in seclusion for an hour after which another colleague took over. Staff did not always introduce themselves to the patient when they arrived or say goodbye when they left, and in this respect, they did not see their behaviour as problematic. Few patients also commented on how they did not like being watched in seclusion by staff that they did not know.

Managing racial abuse

The distancing of staff from the patient in seclusion because of the awkwardness of not wanting to directly look at them is, according to Levinas (2006), linked to the exposure of weakness and vulnerability of face-to-face looking. He refers to the "face" as a term for the other person and believes that it is the opposition of the face which results in the feeling of shame. Therefore, for staff, the awkwardness of looking at the patient in seclusion is linked to their discomfort about looking at them in this intense way. Clegg (2012) suggests that awkwardness is an emotion that people experience when they feel threatened that they might not be accepted by others. However, managing their feelings of awkwardness was not the only reason why some staff preferred watching patients in seclusion using CCTV monitors. On few occasions, when doing fieldwork observations of patients in seclusion, several black staff also chose to close the blinds covering the seclusion observation panel, preferring to use the CCTV monitor exclusively to watch the patient in seclusion. These staff, who either knew the patient or had been told about the patient, claimed that the patient had either been disrespectful to them or other black staff by being racially abusive. For these staff, staying out of sight of the patient enabled them to carry out their job of doing observation without having to deal with the emotional aspect of hearing racial abuse.

This use of cameras provided relief from patient abuse as it enabled black staff to remain anonymous, where they recognised that the watchful gaze also involved accepting that such abuse was part of doing the job. Gallagher (2014: 1) draws on Levinas to claim that the "face is characterised by proximity and distance" and that the closeness of the face "demands a response that could range from a passionate kiss to a punch, or some less extreme or more polite behaviour of moving away or asking for space". As Van Rompay et al. (2009: 62) add, "the presence of others can be seen as a social force, affecting feelings, cognitions, and, to some degree, behaviours". In these circumstances, the closing down of face-to-face encounter while undertaking the job required of them which is to monitor the patient in seclusion, some black staff used the mediation of CCTV to purposefully create a distance between them and the patient. This was so that they could manage their own emotions and protect themselves from racial abuse by the patient.

The boredom of seclusion monitoring

While some authors have examined the emotive effects of surveillance on those being surveilled (see, for example, Koskela, 2000, 2012), less has been said about the emotive effects on those people doing surveillance, especially face-to-face or in-person surveillance. Ellis et al. (2013), for example, describe how surveillance has been theorised to evoke feelings of suspicion, while Koskela (2000) describes how those under surveillance can experience a range of emotions such as anger, guilt and fearfulness. The detachment of staff from the patient in seclusion was also expressed in how a number of them felt about doing seclusion observation. Most staff found it a boring and tedious activity because often there was very little happening. Smith (2007: 292) suggests that CCTV operators are "intensely exposed to the *emotional* control" of camera images that they are watching and as a result can become bored, frustrated and can feel guilt, sadness and anxiety.

> Field note 009: *"observation of the patient is via CCTV monitor – staff says so long as he can hear the patient he does not feel it is necessary to see him … staff spends most time reading his paper, occasionally checking CCTV monitor before recording that he has seen patient. The patient can be heard talking to himself".*

Medical surveillance

Boredom also led some staff to go beyond the role of the watchful nurse to explore the meaning behind patient behaviour through the process of attempting to understand the nature of their mental health condition. Some staff did this because they believed that they were assisting the consultant psychiatrist in their clinical understanding of the patient, especially in assisting the continuing need for seclusion. However, sometimes these staff also wanted to observe patient behaviour because they believed that it would help patients.

> S2: *"It [seclusion] lets us know what they're like cos everybody has their own, I like to think of it as a mask they put on when they come to the communal area, so sort of hide who they are. They might hide how actually ill*

> *they are, they might hide how they're feeling. Erm whereas if you've got someone where they can't see you so they think they're on their own, you can help them figure out who that person is, you can say like you do this and you don't like to do that, whereas in the communal area you don't like to do this and you don't like that. It's quite interesting really. It's like a little observatory".*
>
> S2: "*It's sort of like being a fly on the wall really, watching the monitors, especially in seclusion. Cos if you're not in their eyesight they can't see you, so they think they're on their own. So, you can kind of see someone's behaviour when they think no one's watching them".*

Seclusion monitoring challenges Goffman's (1969) notion of front stage, back stage and off stage behaviours. The unmasking of behaviour inside seclusion is done to expose any behaviour that is not related to the patient's mental disorder. For example, anger as a result of being locked up, anger at a particular staff member, anger at another patient and behaviour related to substance and alcohol misuse. However, as Kutchins and Kirk (1997) observe, the medicalisation of behaviour into mental health conditions embodies a range of behaviours and values that are historically and socially constructed. Although the Mental Health Act Code of Practice (2015: para 26. 107) states that seclusion should not be used as punishment, or because of staff shortage, or as part of a treatment programme, the ability to watch the patient in seclusion without any hindrance allowed some staff to speculate about patient behaviour. Therefore, the seclusion room did become an observatory, where Foucault claims that the "appetite for medicine" results in the appeal of psychiatric experts who then pass "therapeutic" sentences and periods of rehabilitation through imprisonment or incarceration (1979: 304). Inside seclusion, the cameras were less effective as a panoptic tool in the disciplining of patient behaviour. Instead, they functioned as a means to learn about patients and their behaviour. Although the initial reason to segregate the patient from other patients had passed, several patients were often left inside seclusion so that staff could observe other behaviours in order to feel satisfied that the patient would not become aggressive once seclusion had ended.

Depersonalising patients

Levinas (2006) claims that a true relationship can only be ethical when it is demonstrated in the face-to-face encounter. For some staff, distancing themselves from patients in seclusion by choosing to watch them using the CCTV monitor did not always sit comfortably with the role of the watchful nurse. For these staff, CCTV was not a helpful tool in doing seclusion observations. They felt that relying on CCTV monitoring meant that staff lost an opportunity to engage with patients at a time when they were acutely unwell and perhaps needed more attention. These staff also believed that even when patients are at their worst, for example, wiping their faeces around the seclusion room walls, referred to by staff as "dirty protest", they were still wanting human contact. Some patients agreed with this and stated that they felt ignored by staff so that when they asked for things like a book, drink, towel and clean clothes, they believed their requests were not taken seriously. Few patients described seclusion as akin to prison and referred it to as "*segregation zone*", "*the blocks*" or "*prison cell*" (P1). These patients believed that staff preferred to view them via the cameras because they were frightened of them.

Inside the ward, staff generally tended to perceive patients as a collective body. This sometimes extended to how they also perceived patients when they were in seclusion. Inside seclusion patients have nowhere to hide and everything to do with their behaviour and body is exposed. When they come out of the shower, for example, and are naked, this exposure is not just viewed by staff directly responsible for observing them in the seclusion lobby area. Staff in the ward office, and anyone else who is present in the office, can also view the patient's naked body through the ward office CCTV monitor. This constant visibility of the patient body in seclusion also resulted in the de-sensitisation of some staff's attitude towards patients:

> Field note 029: "*One of the staff (female) looking at the screen [CCTV monitor in the ward office] says 'she's taking her clothes off'. This prompts another member of staff (female) to look at the CCTV monitor … The other staff tells me … 'she settles down in between reviews but when we go in there to do a review, she attacks us. It means she's unpredictable. I don't mind what she says, you know, she calls me a bitch and it's like sticks and stones may break my bones and that. No, it's more she lunges forward to attack us'. At this point a male colleague enters the ward office and the staff talking to me says 'yeah (she laughs) she's [meaning the patient] really got a thing you know for x [names the male staff]. Last time we did a nursing review she said she wanted us to all get out of the [seclusion] room so that she can fuck x'. Male staff nurse turns red and looks embarrassed while the other two staff laugh*".

During this discussion, the female patient was topless, and neither of the female staff who were talking about her and looking at the CCTV monitor thought it appropriate to turn the monitor off or reduce its size so that it was difficult to see. Their conversation also prompted the male member of staff who had walked into the room to look at the monitor. Rosenhan describes how he and the pseudopatients in his study were depersonalised in similar ways inside mental health wards.

> At times, depersonalisation reached such proportions that pseudopatients had the sense they were invisible, or at least unworthy of account. Upon being admitted, I and other pseudopatients took the initial physical

examinations in a semipublic room, where staff members went about their own business as if we were not there.

(Rosenhan, 1973: 256)

As a nurse-judge, the normalising gaze in the humour of the two staff is reflected in the disinhibited behaviour and actions of the patient in seclusion who must be undermined to justify the incarceration (Foucault, 1979). These encounters also undermine the fundamental characteristics of the therapeutic gaze, which is not about judging but protecting.

CCTV and staying connected

Being accountable

The availability of the cameras constantly streaming images of patients and staff into the ward office CCTV monitors meant that staff, even when they were in the ward office involved in administration activities, were always aware of their primary function as the vigilant, watchful observer. Staff kept an eye on CCTV monitors as a matter of habit in the event of being ready for any potential disturbances arising inside the ward which needed their attention. Here, cameras were not used to distance themselves from patients but to stay connected with them and the ward environment. Although there is an element to also maintain social order inside the ward by being always ready for potential disturbances, the cameras were not the only device in the ward which could alert staff to potential conflict inside it. All staff, for example, were required to wear a personal alarm when inside the ward, whether they were in the ward office or communal areas of the ward. These were likely to be far more effective in alerting other staff about any dangers or attacks inside the ward than the occasional, random watching of CCTV monitors inside the ward office. Therefore, whilst staff justified watching the monitors as a means to identify trouble, they looked at the monitors mostly because they wanted to stay connected to the ward environment.

> S14: "*If I'm on the computers and I'm opposite them I regularly look up at them to see what's happening, especially if I'm in charge and I'm in the office a lot, then I can see where staff are, I can see where the patients are um and I've got a rough idea about what's happening on the ward*".

These non-specific glances did occasionally capture an event happening inside the ward. Below, an occasional gaze quickly turns into a situation that requires action as the looks between two patients draw attention to the monitor.

> Field note 102: "*One staff glances up to the monitor and says, 'is that man sitting on the lap of another man?' They both come closer to the monitor.*

They decide it might be two men behaving inappropriately and go out into the communal area to investigate further. I watch on the screen. One staff stands back while the other speaks with the patients. Both staff return, and I ask if everything is okay. One staff tells me 'It's okay. It's two women comforting each other'".

Staying connected with the ward environment was therefore not just about keeping an eye on patients. It was also about normalising their behaviour.

Managing anxiety and nurse observations

There were several reasons why staff sometimes believed that it was better not to be directly engaged with patients but to watch them from a distance or to do discrete watching. Below, S10 describes how he used the CCTV monitor in the ward office to watch a patient whom he believed was attempting to outsmart him by finding areas in the ward to hide from him. A situation that may previously have raised anxiety because the patient was out of sight became a playful encounter because he knew where she was.

> S10: *"She thought I weren't watching but you try and sort of be, sort of pretty relaxed about it type of thing and she thought I was a bit too relaxed. I knew where she went and I could see it. She ran down the bottom of the corridor and hid by the back door … but I know there's a camera there so I thought I'm just gonna leave you there cos she thinks that, so I just stood in the office I could see where she was and I could see her on the camera, I could see what she was doing and she thought, she said oh you lost me then. I said I was watching you on the camera I knew where you was all the time".*

Staff's anxiety was also related to ensuring that they were not crowding the patient. Below, S11 and S20 describe scenarios in which they recognise that they need to maintain a distance and at the same time keep an eye on patients. Here, cameras inside the visitor room and outside the ward periphery area are used by the staff as a means of creating distance whilst still allowing them to maintain a watchful stance over patients.

> S11: *"… like with x [patient] and her husband cos they go into the activity room. Instead of standing outside and making them feel … annoyed … it's a private meeting you know … but even though we're stood outside the door, it's still annoying … So instead of doing that we stand in the office and watch [CCTV monitor]".*
>
> S20: *"… say we had a patient erm who was absconding risk, and we were trying to graduate their leave, and we took a bit of a risk and we said why don't you go and have some time out at the front of the building for 15*

minutes erm initially. What we have done in the past is unobtrusively observe them via the CCTV [CCTV monitor in the ward office] so it kind of gives us and them a bit of space, rather than you know be watching them".

This discreet watching was beneficial to staff and patients. It was beneficial to staff because it allowed them to manage their anxiety as they could still keep an eye on the patient. It was beneficial to patients because it allowed them to get on with activities inside the ward. For example, meeting with their visitor privately and by demonstrating to staff that they are ready to leave the ward by showing that they can control their urge to run away when they were outside the building. Several staff believed the cameras were a benefit because they allowed more freedom for patients in the ward. This freedom is expressed in discreet watching which allows the patient to move around the ward without staff having to follow them and to be inside their bedroom without being disturbed.

S23: *"You can still observe someone without physically being there which is amazing, cos I think this unit ... which is locked, there is no independency whatsoever. You have to ask for every single thing, you know things that you need, then having someone follow you all the time, it's not very nice, isn't it? It's just taking all of your privacy and all of your dignity".*

S24: *"So if you come in you don't have to wake them up. Turn it on, see what they are doing and listen to them breathing rather than disturb them because sleep is very important in mental health and if you keep disturbing them it sort of defeats the objective ... So it's got its benefits".*

CCTV as an extra member of staff

CCTV as a helper

The cameras, according to staff, had several potential benefits. For example, they allowed them to occasionally intervene faster in a given situation because the incident had been seen on the CCTV monitor. The combination of visibility of the ward areas from the ward office window panels and the cameras meant that staff could easily observe large parts of the ward, from the ward office. This was especially helpful when the ward was short-staffed or when the staff team took breaks. Also, the cameras' ability to allow nursing staff, who were in charge of the ward, to maintain contact with the ward environment meant that some staff perceived the cameras as akin to having an extra staff member inside it.

S3: *"... it's [CCTV] like having an extra member of staff sometimes cos you can predict it [violent situation] before it happens, you can observe and then intervene quicker".*

> S8: "*I think you can have like I said eyes in many places, and you know it's almost like a second workforce you know. You know there's that old saying erm a thousand men holding the sky never got tired, share the workload and then that way, cos if you're looking all the time at something you do get fatigue and you can't always be checking and it's almost like a second workforce. The camera never lies*".

> S12: "*... it's our job to stay around the patient so that can be done, maybe need err five staff but maybe when you have a camera, we can release one or two, that's an option*".

Using the cameras for nurse observations

The cameras' ability to allow staff to easily view large parts of the ward also meant that staff used them as a shortcut to locating patients. Previously, these staff they may have had to venture out into the ward and physically seek out patients. Therefore, they saw using the cameras as similar to asking a colleague when they last saw the patient but better because they could see the patient in location. For these staff, it was also a quick and efficient way of doing nurse observations because they could easily see the patient on CCTV monitors and those areas that were visible from the ward office windows. This also meant they did not need to make face-to-face contact with them. The seeking out and observation of patients using cameras also meant that during a busy shift, they were not distracted by patients. This would be likely if they ventured into the ward to do face-to-face observations.

> S10: "*Or, if I can't find whoever's on level 2 [observation] because they're right down at the other end of the building. I'll try and see if I can find them on the camera*".

> S8: "*So say if somebody is on 5-minute observation checks, so every 5 minutes we need to check them and err say you've got two or three [patients] at the same time and you're in the office and you can see perhaps a couple of people in the day area, you can see one person on the camera, then you've seen them all you know they're safe*".

> S9: "*If we can, the ones that we can see on camera we would tick em off and it would be the ones we haven't seen we would then go physically and check them*".

Lyon suggests that in a post-Panoptical world, people can "slip away, escaping to unreachable realms". He believes that this is because the post-Panoptical world favours mobility over a mutual engagement (Lyon in Bauman and Lyon, 2013: 4). Most staff identified the benefits of CCTV in the context of doing their job inside the ward as opposed to how doing the job, using the cameras, benefitted patients. Therefore, it was the ability of the cameras to function as an efficient extra pair of eyes, or their flexibility to locate patients easily, or their ability to manage staffing levels inside the ward, which elevated their position from being a piece of equipment or technology to the position of "staff". Ellul (1964: vi) describes how these behaviours or ways of using technology become rationalised. He uses the phrase "*technique*" to describe how behaviour that is "spontaneous and unreflective" is converted into behaviour that is "deliberate and rationalized".

Nurse observation practice inside the ward was often performed as a perfunctory activity. Fieldwork observations inside all three wards suggested that there was not much variation in how this activity was conducted. For example, nurse observations inside all three PICUs involved staff viewing or looking at the patient and either manually ticking boxes on a sheet of paper (which were later recorded onto electronic patient records by administrative staff), or on a computerised electronic tablet. Most staff when doing nurse observations spent little time talking to patients. If anything was said, it was generally to let the patient know that they were doing observations. Staff also carried a clipboard or computer tablet with them so that the patient could see that observation was happening. This aspect of nurse observations was noteworthy for two reasons. By visibly carrying the clipboard or computer tablet, staff gave the message that they were busy carrying out a task and therefore unavailable to the patient. Second, the significance of the clipboard or computer tablet was that they could show (possibly) the patient, but other staff around them that they had been accountable.

This behaviour by staff was also apparent when they used cameras to locate patients inside the ward while carrying out nurse observations. At these times, fieldwork observations revealed staff standing in front of the ward office CCTV monitor, looking intently at it and ticking off patients that they had seen on their clipboard or computer tablet showing anyone else in the ward office that they had done nurse observations. In this way, staff perceived the cameras as a way of improving the task of nurse observations inside the ward. This is because there was no need for them to venture out into all parts of the ward as some patients could easily be viewed through the glass panels in the ward office and others could be accounted for via the CCTV monitor. Also, it allowed other staff in the office, usually qualified nursing staff, to see that they had done their nurse monitoring task and had been accountable for ensuring that each patient was safe. Peplau (1988) suggested that at the heart of mental health nursing was the nurse–patient relationship. Since she analysed the importance of this relationship in the recovery of patients, there have been several other models of health care based on person-centred or relational approaches (Freeth, 2007). These approaches to mental health nursing care become threatened as nursing care starts to become constructed around viewing the patient and not engaging with the patient. In this way, the pastoral role becomes less favoured over efficiency, where even therapeutic activities are systemised and mechanised so that patients have set times to talk about what is bothering them, with set staff (their key worker on that shift) and often inside a ward environment which can sometimes feel as S2 below describes as "pent-up".

> S2: *"whereas here when I came here it was very pent-up, signed out, you watch them all the time and then they showed me all the cameras".*

It is these mechanistic activities and specific ways of doing even person-centred practice that places the patient under increasing supervision. What is lost in these performance or tick-box-related practices is why nurses do observations and what benefits patients gain from nurse observations. Ellul's notion of *technique*, therefore, is not limited to CCTV, it is also "the *totality of methods rationally arrived at and having absolute efficiency* ... in *every* field of human activity" (Ellul, 1964: xxv). In this respect, Ellul believes there is no restraint on the rules of *technique* because the hospital as an institution is also "orientated towards 'performance' and *technique* is regarded as the prime instrument of performance" (Ellul, 1964: vi).

Ellul's (1964) theoretical analysis of *technique* provides an understanding of how the cameras can easily become a by-product of efficiency, resulting in his claim that is the political doctrine of what is useful that dominates over what is good. Furthermore, Ellul also claimed that it is rational technology combined with scientific expertise and objectivity that has provided the pre-requisite for new technologies to become not only a tool inside the ward but also the fabric of the ward where staff believe that they could not function the same without it. The establishment and acceptance of CCTV as a necessary tool within the context of the ward has to happen alongside the goals of the staff at an operational level as well as at an organisational level. Ellul claims that it is when people learn to ignore the mechanisms of *technique* that technology becomes most efficient. He referred to this process as social plasticity (Ellul, 1964). Social plasticity inside the ward was demonstrated by the fact that some staff perceived the cameras as indispensable.

> S6: *"The cameras are so part of the ward and they're there cos they're needed".*
>
> S20: *"... if we didn't have it [CCTV], it's hard to imagine what it would be like if it [CCTV] had to be taken away".*

The cameras as (an unreliable) colleague

Warnick (2007: 326), when examining the ethics of CCTV use inside schools, believed that one of the reasons why the use of cameras inside schools caused little disagreement within communities was because they were perceived as "a natural extension of a watchful and observant school official". For some staff, unlike human colleagues, whose account of what happened in a given situation might be sketchy, open to interpretation and potentially judgemental, the cameras were seen as more reliable in their account of what happened in a given situation. In this way, the cameras were also perceived as a better ally, especially where a staff's behaviour was under question or suspicion. In these situations, staff also perceived the cameras as an extended member of staff, whose reliability transcended "the vagaries of memory" and could also potentially provide an accurate account of an incident (Warnick, 2007: 326).

> S10: *"But the thing is though, your anxieties go up! And if they [managers] had just gone and turned around and said alright let's just rewind the camera, oh x [mentions own name] yes you did catch her in the throat accidentally, but I didn't anyway, but it takes out all that".*
>
> S13: *"So it's not going to be just, if you're having to, for instance, a patient attacking you it's not only you, your, you know, your opinion and the patient, you've got that as proof then that they did attack you".*
>
> S17: *"But you don't always remember either. So, there is that element where actually the camera, but the camera doesn't lie".*

However, as well as protecting them, some staff also recognised that the cameras could expose their practices to others which could result in gossip.

> S12: *"... any small thing what's happened ... staff will go and check on the camera ... then the rumour will start to spread aww this happened ... everyone [senior nursing staff] can access a camera [CCTV monitor], so they will go and check, they will tell other people what exactly happened, who did what, so that's a little uncomfortable sometimes".*

However, unlike human colleagues, where the likelihood is that gossip would probably dissipate quickly, with CCTV recordings, there was the potential for the matter to remain longer in people's memories. Those staff who had access to recordings were able to view the footage over and over again and present their version of an event each time. Thus, events at times were both blown out of proportion and also remained in the memories of staff much longer. Also, while staff made a judgement about whether they should report another colleague's misdemeanours, the cameras were not limited by such conventions. Below, S20 describes the limitations of visual footage.

> S20: *"I think sometimes footage can be, can, can portray something that it didn't feel like in the moment".*

CCTV and peer surveillance

> Field note 004: *"Two female staff looking at the monitor. Both get annoyed because the patient and patient visitor are kissing. One staff tells me 'they could be passing anything' (meaning that the patient's visitor could be*

> *passing drugs to the patient via kissing). Staff member says that the staff nurse (qualified nurse in charge) should speak with the agency staff who is monitoring the visit, that patients should not be making contact".*

Post-Panoptical analysis of surveillance suggests that the addition of CCTV cameras inside the ward expands to those people who were not previously the focus of attention. The above field note is of two staff critically assessing an agency worker's performance during the monitoring of a visit between a patient and their visitor. The visitor room has a CCTV camera located inside it, which can be viewed from the ward office. However, unlike the seclusion area which has a lobby next to the seclusion room with a CCTV monitor, there is no CCTV monitor directly outside the visitor room. The agency staff monitoring the visit is sat outside the visitor room which has a large window panel that looks into the room. Therefore, the agency worker may not have been able to see all interaction between the patient and the visitor in the same way as the cameras allowed the staff inside the ward office to view the visitor room.

Sewell (2012: 304) describes how subordinates perform peer-to-peer scrutiny in the workplace and in this way perform a form of horizontal surveillance, through critiquing behaviours that may or may not be "organisationally appropriate". He suggests that there is a difference between the embodied mutual gaze of peers and the disembodied gaze embedded in technology. During this encounter, the comment and tone of speech used by the two staff watching the CCTV monitor were abrupt and harsh. Although they were watching the patient and his visitor, the conversation between them was about the agency staff who was not visible on camera. Therefore, each action by the patient or his visitor which they perceived was a breach of ward rules was emphasised to show that the agency worker was not competent at her job. For example, the patient had a bottled drink with him, and this made them question whether he had taken it from the ward or whether the visitor has had passed him the bottle, which might have alcohol inside it. These comments led to a conversation where they described the inefficiency of most agency staff whom they believed were not committed to the job, and whom they perceived as "free-riders" (Sewell, 2012: 305).

This critical approach by staff towards their colleagues was also evident in interviews with staff where the cameras had captured certain behaviours. Below, S11 is angry with a manager because he had breached the rules of the ward by allowing a stranger into the air-lock space without checking the person's credentials. S8 and S24 are questioning the efficacy of agency and bank staff whom they believe are less committed to the job and are likely to take longer breaks, sleep on the job and so on. Therefore, the core staff team were often suspicious of some managers who were not regular visitors to the ward and of bank and agency staff, whom they believed were not as committed to watching out for patients as they were.

S11: *"The manager allowed that person ... onto the ward, never thought nothing of it. So, I go out to the airlock then and there's this chap stood there, Indian chap stood there I recognised him, and I said can I help you? And he said I'm looking for doctor ... whoever it is, looking for the Consultant next door. I asked him who'd let him in ... I said can you, can you stop here [in the airlock space] because he had no ID, no nothing. I'm fuming a bit now because who's let him on? We don't know him ... found out that this person was, is a patient who'd just got out of prison for beating his wife up ...".*

S8: *"We do have a lot of agency workers yeah because we cannot predict the amount of staff that we need from a week to week basis, so that's expected. Erm sometimes you get people that take longer breaks than they should, or they might fall asleep at work, or they might not know the protocols or procedures around ... performing restraint ...".*

S24: *"... sometimes on night-shifts ... staff can't take forty-winks knowing that, that thing [CCTV] is watching me ... so if anything, it encourages people to be on the floor [in the communal area]".*

CCTV and the negative categorisation of patients

Jenkins (2012: 160) suggests that identity is not only about self-identification and is "an interplay between internal *self-identification* – which can be individual or collective – and external *categorisation* by others". Inside the ward, patients are categorised according to their mental disorder and (often risky) related behaviour. Some of these behaviours are at times linked to fight or flight behavioural responses (Cannon, 1915). Therefore, some patients were perceived to be "fight" risk and likely to hurt other people, and some were perceived as a "flight" risk, who sought ways to escape the ward. Below, S23 describes the importance of recognising the effects of patients who are highly charged.

S23: *"people (patients) when they are sometimes really unwell they can sometimes be really scared, then you know, adrenalin is coming in they can do more than they would normally if you know what I mean. Like jumping over the fences and stuff, which that fence is quite high you wouldn't normally do it, would you but I think when adrenalin is pumping in it's different".*

This heightened level of fear of being inside the ward and their attempts to escape the ward led some staff to attribute certain superhuman qualities to these patients. Below, S7 and S9 use terminologies such as "Hulk" and "Houdini" to describe patient behaviour. These and similar terms became associated with patients even though once they had settled into the ward they were no longer involved in absconding behaviour. The recorded images of the patient escaping the ward or attempting to escape the ward and viewed by many staff, often as part of learning from an incident reinforce these stereotypes.

> S7: *"It's mainly an absconsion thing, cos from both the gardens people [patients] can get in and out. We've had a patient climb up onto the roof from the garden … cos we used to have table and chairs set in there, they're all weighted down but somehow it [patient] became like Hulk and managed to pick the chair up and managed to put it on top of the table and managed to climb up onto the roof".*
>
> S9: *"actually someone [patient] was a very, was a Houdini, and actually climbed through the windows up in the ceiling …"*

This was also the case for patients who had been aggressive or violent. Inside one research site, a male patient was left in seclusion for 20 days because the clinical team were afraid to let him out due to his violent behaviour associated with his previous admission to the ward, which was over a year ago. During this previous admission, he had badly damaged the seclusion room, and while he was inside the ward, he also physically assaulted a member of staff. While these two incidences were very serious, any decision-making about his current care was heavily influenced by his behaviour during his previous admission. The likelihood of being left in seclusion with no idea of when he would be released meant that the patient was often angry, verbally abusive, threatening violence towards staff and kicking doors and panels inside the seclusion room. The categorisation by the staff of this patient as a dangerous and violent individual meant that even those staff who did not know him were fearful of him. The continuous availability of CCTV footage of this patient in seclusion, to staff in the ward office, exacerbated the situation because the constant visual image of the patient on the CCTV monitor in the ward office tended to prompt negative discussions about him.

> Field note 026: *"Patient x still in seclusion (13th day). When I walk into the ward office there are several staff clustered around CCTV monitor watching patient x. Conversation lasts for about 25 mins. Staff talking about how patient x has been racially abusive to black staff when they have been involved in seclusion monitoring. During this time staff look at the CCTV monitor. Staff are talking about management decision to have 3 staff in seclusion area and leaving the seclusion room door open. Staff are concerned about their safety and the mood is low. This is supposed to happen later today, but managers are in a discussion about whether this should happen or not. Some staff adamant that if they are asked to monitor patient x they will refuse. Staff also talking about contacting their union reps".*

Marx (1998: 180) poses the question of whether surveillance technology is "likely to create precedents that will lead to its application in an undesirable way". Whilst it is not definitive, there was a suggestion that the availability of CCTV footage streaming continuously inside the ward office did prompt negative discussions about particular patients, simply because they were more visible. This visibility went beyond simply watching or keeping an eye on them; it also led to them being categorised as high risk and dangerous, where the focus is on their behaviour. Below, S22 demonstrates how patients become reduced to their behaviour and actions inside the ward.

> S22: "*So you can have a look, say okay so this person's [patient] a puncher or this person [patient] kicks when you take him in this position or this person [patient] is particularly targeting these people or, and just kind of have a look for general patterns and things like that*".

Conclusion

In this chapter, I have drawn on Winner's (1977) theorisation of function creep and Marx's (1988) surveillance creep to highlight how the camera use was extended beyond the recommendation made by NAPICU. The central theme of this chapter is that the presence of the cameras and the availability of CCTV footage raised staff expectations about the violent nature of PICU patients. Worryingly, it also raised expectations about how managers should respond to any violence from patients towards them as staff. Therefore, when evidence of incidents was available on CCTV footage, staff were disappointed when managers or the police did not respond harshly, for example, by prosecution and taking the matter to court. Also, the ability of the cameras to capture evidence of the violent nature of the mental health patient meant that staff wanted more cameras inside the ward, especially hot-spot areas for aggressive behaviour. This focus on the violent nature of the mental health patient influences how therapeutic care is practised inside the ward.

Some key practice implications arising out of this chapter include:

- How the presence of cameras in some parts of the ward has resulted in staff wanting more cameras in all parts of the ward and thereby expanding surveillance.
- How the cameras expose already existing tensions between managers and frontline staff, especially when using the cameras to investigate some staff practices and interventions.
- The reduction in face-to-face contact with patients as the cameras increasingly become the medium by which staff observe patients.
- How the introduction of cameras in certain parts of the ward, such as bedrooms, seclusion room and spaces used by all patients undermines ethical practice.

- How the cameras have the potential to expose women patient bodies in ways which not only undermine ethical practice but also raise serious safeguarding concerns.
- The ability of the cameras to change the balance of care and control inside the ward through the negative categorisation of patients.
- The ability of the cameras to make patients accountable, for their part, in any aggressive and violent behaviour inside the ward.

Chapter 6 will draw together some key theoretical debates arising from this chapter. Chapter 5 examines how patients as a subject of surveillance experience the cameras and the mental health ward.

Bibliography

Ball, K., Canhoto, A., Daniel, E., Dibb, S., Meadows, M. and Spiller, K. (2015). *The Private Security State? Surveillance, Consumer Data and the War on Terror*, Frederiksberg: Copenhagen Business School Press.

Bauman, Z. and Lyon, D. (2013). *Liquid Surveillance*, Cambridge: Polity Press.

Bennett, R., Ramakrishna, V. and Magarity, D. (2011). "Management of disturbed behaviour in a psychiatric intensive care unit: Views of staff on options for intervention," *Journal of Psychiatric Intensive Care Unit*, 7(2): 85–89.

Bijker, W.E. (1995). *Of Bicycles, Bakelites and Bulbs: Towards a Theory of Sociotechnical Change*, Cambridge: MIT Press.

Bowers, L., Jeffrey, D., Bigin, H., Jarrett, M., Simpson, A. and Jones, J. (2008). "Psychiatric intensive care units: A literature review," *International Journal of Social Psychiatry*, 54(1): 56–68.

Cameron, H. (2004). "CCTV and (in)dividuation," *Surveillance and Society*, 2(2/3): 136–144.

Cannon, W.B. (1915). *Bodily Changes in Pain, Hunger, Fear, and Rage*, New York: Appleton-Century-Crofts.

Chambers, M. and Gillard, S. (2005). *Review of CCTV on John Meyer Ward, 19 July 2005 Agenda Item 9, South West London and St George's NHS Mental Health Trust*, South West London and St George's NHS Mental Health Trust Board Meeting, 28 July 2005, London.

Clegg, J. (2012). "Stranger situations: Examining a self-regulatory model of socially awkward encounters," *Group Processes and Intergroup Relations*, 15(6): 693–712.

Collins English Dictionary. (1979). *Collins English Dictionary of the English Language*, London: Collins.

Dahl, J.Y. and Saetnan, A.R. (2009). "'It all happened so slowly' – On controlling function creep in forensic DNA databases," *International Journal of Law, Crime and Justice*, 37: 83–103.

Ellis, D., Tucker, I. and Harper, D. (2013). "The affective atmospheres of surveillance," *Theory and Psychology*, 23(6): 716–731.

Ellul, J. (1964). *The Technological Society*, New York: Vintage Books.

Freeth, R. (2007). *Humanising Psychiatry and Mental Health Care: The Challenge of the Person-Centered Approach*, Oxford: Radcliffe Publishing.

Foucault, M. (1979). *Discipline and Punish: The Birth of the Prison*, New York: Vintage.
Foucault, M. (2009). *Security, Territory, Population: Lectures at the Collège de France 1977–1978*, edited by Michel Senellart and translated by Graham Burchell, Basingstoke: Palgrave.
Gallagher, S. (2014). "In your face: Transcendence in embodied interaction," *Frontiers of Human Neuroscience*, 8: 1–6. Available online: www.frontiersin.org [accessed 20 May 2019].
Garland, D. (2001). *The Culture of Control: Crime and Social Order in Contemporary Society*, Oxford: Oxford University Press.
Gilburt, H., Rose, D. and Slade, M. (2008). "The importance of relationships in mental health care: A qualitative study of service users' experiences of psychiatric hospital admission in the UK," *BMC Health Service Research*, 8(92): 1–12. Available online: www.biomedcentral.com/1472-6963/8/92 [accessed 8 May 2019].
Goffman, E. (1961). *Asylums: Essays on the Social Situation of Mental Patients and Other Inmates*, New York: Anchor Books.
Goffman, E. (1969). *The Presentation of the Self in Everyday Life,* Great Britain: Allen Lane, Penguin Press.
Haggerty, K.D. (2012). "Surveillance, crime and the police," in K. Ball, K.D. Haggerty and D. Lyon (eds), *Routledge Handbook of Surveillance Studies*, London: Routledge, pp. 235–243.
Hope, A. (2009). "CCTV, school surveillance and social control," *British Educational Research Journal*, 35(6): 891–907.
Jenkins, R. (2012). "Identity, surveillance and modernity: Sorting out who's who," in K. Ball, K.D. Haggerty and D. Lyon (eds), *Routledge Book of Surveillance Studies*, London: Routledge, pp. 159–166.
Karban, K. (2011). *Social Work and Mental Health*, Cambridge: Polity Press.
Koskela, H. (2000). "The gaze without eyes: Video-surveillance and the changing nature of urban space," *Progress in Human Geography*, 24(2): 243–265.
Koskela, H. (2012). " 'You shouldn't wear that body': The problematic of surveillance and gender," in K. Ball, K.D. Haggerty and D. Lyon (eds), *Routledge Handbook of Surveillance Studies*, London: Routledge, pp. 49–56.
Kutchins, H. and Kirk, S.A. (1997). *Making Us Crazy: DSM – The Psychiatric Bible and the Creation of Mental Disorders*, London: Constable.
Levinas, E. (2006). *Humanism of the Other*, translated by N. Poller and Introduction by R.A. Cohen, Urbana and Chicago: University of Illinois Press.
Marx, G.T. (1988). *Undercover: Police Surveillance in America*, Berkley: University of California.
Marx, G.T. (1998). "Ethics for the new surveillance," *Information Society*, 14: 171–185.
McCahill, M. and Norris, C. (2003). "Victims of surveillance," in P. Davis, V. Jupp and P. Francis (eds), *Victimisation: Theory, Research and Policy*, Basingstoke: Palgrave Macmillan, pp. 121–147.
National Association of Psychiatric Intensive and Low Secure Care Units (NAPICU). (2014). *National Minimum Standards for Psychiatric Intensive Care in General Adult Services*, East Kilbride: NAPICU International Press.
National Association of Psychiatric and Intensive and Low Secure Care Units (NAPICU) and NHS Clinical Commissioners. (2016). *Guidance for Commissioners of Psychiatric Intensive Care Units (PICU)*, East Kilbride: NAPICU International Press.

National Health Service (NHS) England. (2010). *Serious Incident Framework: Supporting Learning to Prevent Recurrence*, NHS England Patient Safety Domain, Skipton House, London.

Norris, C. and Armstrong, G. (1999). *The Maximum Surveillance Society: The Rise of CCTV*, London: Routledge.

Peplau, H.E. (1988). "The art and science of nursing: Similarities, differences, and relations," *Nursing Science Quarterly*, 1: 8–15.

Quirk, A., Lelliot, P. and Seale, C. (2006). "A permeable institution: An ethnographic study of three acute psychiatric wards in London," *Social Science and Medicine*, 63: 2105–2117.

Rosenhan, D.L. (1973). "On being sane in insane places," *Science*, 179: 250–258.

Saverimuttu, A. and Lowe, T. (2000). "Aggressive incidents on a psychiatric intensive care unit," *Nursing Standard*, 23(14): 33–36.

Sewell, G. (2012). "Organisation, employees and surveillance," in K. Ball, K.D. Haggerty and D. Lyon (eds), *Routledge Handbook of Surveillance Studies*, London: Routledge, pp. 303–312.

Smith, G.J.D. (2007). "Exploring relations between watchers and watched in control(led) systems: Strategies and tactics," *Surveillance and Society*, 4(4): 280–313.

Van Rompay, T.J.L., Vonk, D. and Fransen, M. (2009). "The eye of the camera: Effects of security cameras on prosocial behaviour," *Environment and Behaviour*, 41(1): 60–74.

Verbeek, P.P. (2016). "Toward a theory of technological mediation: A program for post phenomenological research," in J.K.B.O Friis and R.C. Crease (eds), *Technoscience and Postphenomenology: The Manhattan Papers*, London: Lexington Books, pp. 189–204.

Warnick, B.R. (2007). "Surveillance cameras in schools: An ethical analysis," *Harvard Educational Review*, 77: 317–393.

Warr, J., Page, M. and Crossen-White, H. (2005). *The Appropriate Use of Closed Circuit Television (CCTV) in a Secure Unit*, Study undertaken by Montpellier Unit and Bournemouth University, England.

Winner, L. (1977). *Autonomous Technology: Technics-Out-Of-Control as a Theme for Political Thought*, Cambridge: MIT Press.

Chapter 5

Patient and staff experiences of CCTV

Introduction

Chapter 3 has identified the various reasons for camera introduction inside the ward. Chapter 4 has highlighted some of the ways that camera use has established itself into everyday mental healthcare practices inside the ward. This chapter aims to analyse how patients attach meaning to, interpret and experience cameras inside the ward. Patients are not the only people inside the ward who are subject to camera surveillance. Staff are also watched by the cameras. Some staff views have been highlighted in this chapter, especially their awareness of cameras and their knowledge about them. However, the main focus of the chapter is about the patient experience of cameras.

This chapter is divided into four broad sections. The first and second parts include patient and staff awareness of cameras, how they felt about the cameras and what they know about the cameras, including why they believed the cameras were inside the ward. The third and fourth parts are linked to patient responses to the cameras and their attempts to resist camera surveillance.

Background

The patient's worldview of the ward is influenced by several interrelated factors. For instance, the ward environment is perceived as a temporary measure. However, the nature of the ward is such that patients do not have a discharge date and neither do they know what they need to achieve to facilitate their discharge. This creates a sense of unpredictability and uncertainty which for some patients can be both frightening and threatening. The hierarchical nature of the ward, where they have little say in their recovery, means that patients are placed in a subordinate position to staff. In the context of the ward, patients also recognise that it is their consultant psychiatrist who has the power to discharge them from the ward and ultimately their detention. Therefore, they are always looking at means and ways of influencing their consultant psychiatrist who is often absent from the ward. The ward

DOI: 10.4324/9781003179306-5

environment becomes an unpredictable place where patients often struggle to settle down into a routine and where they have to learn to live in a restricted and locked space.

When people enter the locked environment of a prison, they know that they are in such an environment because they have been accused of committing a crime. Inside a mental health ward, patients are not always sure why they are kept in a locked environment. The act of being locked inside a ward without knowing when and how they can influence their discharge in itself caused some patients to feel stressed. Unlike the prison, where it is possible to have an end date for the prison sentence, this was not the case inside the mental health ward. It was this not knowing that made the hospital a panoptic machine (Foucault, 2008). During fieldwork observations, several patients expressed their frustration of being inside the ward by kicking furniture and doors because staff could not tell them why they could not be discharged from it. Also, while attempting to recover from their own mental health condition, patients had to cope with their feelings of being locked up, be around other patients who have a mental health condition and cope with other patient's frustrations. This prompted some patients to feel that they needed to be constantly vigilant while they were inside the ward, looking out for other patients (and occasionally staff) who might be a threat to them. This made daily living inside the ward a precarious process, where the patient has to manage their emotions and also be on the constant lookout for others, as getting into an altercation with them may result in prolonging their stay inside the ward.

Ball (2009: 640) suggests that surveillance literature has assumed that "surveillance has consequences for the individual" and that what is lacking is a better theoretical analysis of the surveilled subject. She has highlighted the concept of "exposure", alongside the notion of privacy as a potential starting point in the analysis of those people who are subject to surveillance. Previous research data chapters have shown that the concept of privacy inside restricted ward spaces has produced challenges for managers and staff, especially in the management of patient dignity. This chapter follows this through to examine how the lack of privacy and the continuous process of being looked at, impacts the patient experience of CCTV surveillance inside the ward. This examination of how patients, as subjects of CCTV surveillance, respond to being under surveillance has to have as its starting point an understanding of patient's awareness of CCTV cameras, and what knowledge they have about the cameras, to understand what meaning they attach to them. This meaning in the context of the mental health ward is different from other situations because the nature of the patient's mental health condition can also affect how they respond to cameras inside it. Also, patients know that a key function of the mental health ward is to observe them. Therefore, for them, the cameras have a greater significance. This is because the cameras also provide a vehicle to demonstrate to others that they are ready to be discharged from the ward.

Koskela (2000) believes that looking at how people respond to surveillance can also change the nature of power relations. This is because the lived space inside the ward is looked at not only by those people who control the space but also by those who are looked at. She refers to this as "emotional space" and describes it as space that is "below the threshold at which visibility begins" (Koskela, 2000: 244). Also, Taylor (2014) suggests that subjectivity is not a state that is occupied but is instead an activity that is performed. She draws on Foucault's work to analyse the difference between power and freedom and suggests that engaging in the power of freedom is what keeps power relations dynamic, even when the relationship is not equal. This is because the patient is not in a state of domination in which there are no responses possible. Inside the ward, there were some patients, for example, who refused to take their medication, and in this way, they disrupted the actions of staff. Taylor's (2014) analysis suggests that although the relationship between the patient and staff is not equal, they can still attempt to change their actions even though they may not always be successful.

Awareness of CCTV

Finding out about the cameras

The Information Commissioner's Office Code of Practice for surveillance cameras states that the hospital "must let people know when they are in an area where a surveillance system is in operation" (2017: 37). In all three PICU sites, there was no CCTV signage in the ward or inside the unit to warn patients, staff and any visitors to the ward that CCTV cameras were being used in communal spaces of the ward. Patients and staff tended to find out about the cameras through the research or being told about it by another staff member or patient, or by asking about the cameras, or spotting the cameras in the ward and noticing the CCTV monitors in the ward office.

> P2: *"When you told me. I didn't know. They didn't tell me anything!"*
>
> P3: *"Only from a patient on my first day".*
>
> P4: *"I think I found out last year when I was on x ward. I think they have it in the garden".*
>
> P6: *"… I just noticed the monitor in the office and erm I noticed the, the special cameras are protected erm I wasn't shown. I saw them in the first few days of being here".*
>
> P7: *"No information at all about CCTV on the ward. Nothing".*

No complaints

For both patients and staff, the hierarchical nature of camera use was evident in their belief that they could do nothing about them. When patients were asked what they could do about camera surveillance, most responded with irritation and annoyance. For these patients, it was yet another thing inside the ward over which they had no control.

P4: *"Fuck all".*

P11: *"Bugger all! Nothing. Absolutely nothing. No appeal process. No process of stopping it. They just do what they want".*

P12: *"Err nothing ... Well I haven't been told anything about CCTV and what my rights are or err what my options are with regard to CCTV. I'm not, I've got no idea whether they're recording or not and what happens to the information that they have".*

P6: *"I don't own the ward you know (laughs). There's nothing I can do about it".*

P5: *"Erm well when you're on the ward like this there's not really a great deal of power. Erm you've just gotta sort of discuss with staff your issues and fears and see what they can do to erm to resolve it".*

Similarly, several staffs also believed that they could not do anything about the cameras. These staff felt that they would have no option other than to seek a job elsewhere if they did not like being watched by the cameras, resulting in the loss of potentially good staff from the ward.

S2: *"I think if you don't like being watched then I don't think that this is the place of work for you".*

S8: *"Probably look for another job".*

S15: *"Nothing! There isn't anything I ... I don't think there is anything I could do other than leave".*

S19: *"Work somewhere else I suppose".*

S22: *"Work on a different PICU I guess".*

S24: *"Probably find another job".*

For their part, most managers believed that the lack of complaints from patients and staff about the cameras meant that both patients and staff accepted having cameras inside the ward. Similar to managers, most staff tended to believe that because patients did not actively complain about the cameras, they were accepting of them and were not bothered by them.

S17: *"not in the time I've been here, ever hear a patient complain about it, or verbalise that they weren't happy about it".*

S20: *"I don't think I've ever come across anyone who's gone around going switch them off ... and that has been that erm distressed by it".*

However, when patients have raised it as an issue, staff have not necessarily understood why any patient might want to object to their use or be concerned about them. P12 (below) is talking about staff response to camera use in his bedroom, which he believed staff could view from the CCTV monitor in the office. P14 has been told by the staff to not become too concerned about communal area cameras because their function is limited. These discussions did not address patient anxieties about the use of cameras, which were related to who was looking at the live feeds or recorded footage.

> P12: *"I've had one conversation about the cameras, and I've had to err you know raise it and all she said was that they don't look, they don't look through the cameras from the office".*
>
> P14: *"they said we don't even watch the cameras, they're just recording. It's more of a situation if there's an incident and we can go back. So that kind of relieves the pressure a bit. It's not like there's one guy sitting in the office there looking at the multiscreen going huh there goes x [uses his own name] you know, it's not that way so but I still don't know now who's watching the cameras".*

Part of the territory

Several staff accepted cameras because they expected them as part of their working environment inside a PICU. These staff did not believe that it was unusual to have cameras in the ward, and they saw them as S18 (below) states, coming "*with the territory*". This is because they expected PICUs to be caring for patients who were likely to be highly agitated, experiencing acute symptoms and possibly also under the influence of alcohol or substance use. These patients were perceived as likely to be more disturbed and aggressive because they had either already been violent inside another ward, or they had threatened violence, or they had been violent during a previous admission. Patients were often referred to a PICU when it was not possible to nurse them in other ward environments, such as an acute ward, because their behaviour meant that they needed more intensive support. The normalisation and expectation of the cameras were therefore linked to working in a tough ward environment.

> S2: *"So, I don't think that there's anyone that's bothered by it really, cos they just know it's part of the ward".*
>
> S4: *"If you move everywhere has got CCTV so you could end up with no job".*
>
> S18: *"But yeah if you, if you choose to work in this environment, you choose to be watched all day ... It's just one of those things that comes with the territory of working in a place in, in intensive care".*

Staff were not alone in expecting PICUs to have cameras inside them. Some patients were also not surprised to see the cameras inside the ward. Similar to staff, these patients also associated the presence of cameras with violent behaviours from other patients. These patients accepted that the cameras were there to look out for them and other people.

> P8: *"I'd be very surprised if it didn't a place like this that would be very dangerous. (I: So, you expect there to be cameras here?). Oh god yeah! Definitely!"*
>
> P10: *"The only thing I don't like about it is that I do worry that they're filming us but again I think it's a safety thing, it's for my safety and for everybody's safety on the ward".*

Ward surveillance and normalisation of CCTV

Similar to patients, some staff, especially agency and bank staff, were not told about the cameras inside the ward. Like patients, most of these staff tended to find out about camera use by noticing CCTV monitors in the ward office. Most staff generally expected the ward to have camera surveillance because it was a PICU. However, their expectations about seeing cameras inside the ward were also influenced by camera use outside the hospital, in society. For these staff, the cameras were part of a normal backdrop to everyday life that had minimal impact on them, resulting in them adopting a perspective which, Ellis et al. (2013) claim, takes a pro-surveillance view of the cameras. Webster and Murakami Wood (2009) suggest that it is not the proliferation of technologies that results in the normalisation of surveillance. It is when the emotional, symbolic and cultural domains of society become colonised that normalisation of surveillance occurs. Therefore, these staffs were not shocked or disturbed by the presence of cameras inside the ward and believed them to be a normal part of mental health care.

> S8: *"I saw the cameras so, and I think it was an assumption as well that I made, doing a bit of background reading into psychiatric intensive care units and what have you, so I was sort of, anticipated that".*
>
> S2: *"So I don't think that there's anyone that's bothered by it really, cos they just know it's part of the ward".*
>
> S5: *"I was not surprised that this sort of thing [CCTV] is in place because it's a standard in every hospital I've ever worked. So, for me it was pretty normal".*
>
> S13: *"It was just part of the ward".*

Although most patients had noticed the cameras, they were not always told about them by staff and neither were they given any explanation (written or verbal) as to why they were in the ward. Also, as S22 describes below, most staff did not see the need to let patients know about the cameras. As already identified in Chapter 3, in all three sites, CCTV monitors were mostly visible to patients where they could see the monitors inside the ward office. Therefore, unlike the more common uses of cameras, for example, in open street surveillance and inside shopping malls, where those under surveillance are not always certain about who is watching them, inside the ward, there was no attempt to hide the cameras or the CCTV monitors and patients knew that staff used them to keep an eye on them.

The exposure of the surveilled body through visibility is, and remains, a central aspect of surveillance literature (Haggerty and Ericson, 2007; Lyon, 2007; Elmer, 2012). Foucault's (1979) analysis of the Panopticon has tended to emphasise the visibility of those under surveillance and the unverifiability of those doing surveillance in disciplining behaviour. Inside the ward, patients not only know that they are looked at, but they also know who is looking at them. This is because the openness of the ward offices in all three sites made it easy for patients to see who was inside them. As S22 claims in the quote below, while they might not be telling patients about the use of CCTV cameras inside the ward, they are not attempting to hide them. Similarly, most patients had noticed the cameras for themselves.

> S22: *"I don't think we would directly tell them as part of their kind of erm when they come onto the ward and we show them around and things like that but we're quite happy to point them out if a patients like oh what's this, oh that's a CCTV camera. And obviously our viewing station [CCTV monitors] is visible to them as well … we're not trying to hide it".*
>
> P11: *"No I saw them on the screen. I saw them on the screen in there [meaning CCTV monitors in the ward office]. I saw them on the computers. I saw them on the screen on their computers".*
>
> P12: *"I don't remember being told about it [patient is talking about bedroom camera] but I saw it when I came in. I just, you know it's a big, big black box so I could see it. Yeah no one's had any conversation with me about CCTV".*

"Nothing to hide"

Most staff believed that the cameras did not influence how they did their job inside the ward. The phrase that they had "nothing to hide" and that they often forgot about the cameras once they were in the ward was regularly used to describe their acceptance of cameras (Solove, 2007). Ellis et al. (2013) found that participants in their study initially held very fixed views about surveillance, which when probed further became more fluid, ambivalent and ambiguous. Therefore, the same staff who also believed that the cameras were just part of the ward and were seen but unnoticed, when probed further, admitted that at times the exposure of camera surveillance did make them feel uncomfortable. This discomfort was linked to what other staff might think about their behaviour (peer surveillance), how managers might perceive their actions (performance surveillance) and how those staff, who have an understanding about psychology, because it is a mental health ward, might perceive their actions (behavioural surveillance). These views suggest that several staff did have an awareness of cameras, and this awareness influenced how they behaved inside the ward.

> S8: *"You get very self-conscious about adjusting clothes and you know that kind of thing. And you know that that did worry me a little bit as what will people think of my behaviour, would my behaviour be monitored as well?"*
>
> S9: *"Thinking back on it I would, I would sort of be very cautious of what I was doing when I was in the area of the CCTV camera".*
>
> S12: *"Sometimes I feel a bit uncomfortable some time but that's all".*
>
> S15: *"I don't know what x does. He might look at it all the time". [S15 is talking about the CCTV monitor in the manager's office].*
>
> S20: *"I'm a registered nurse, so I'm constantly mindful of how I portray myself but I'm also aware that I'm in an environment where there's a camera watching me as well".*
>
> S25: *"So I think erm yeah it puts extra pressure on you cos like you have to be absolutely sure".*

Some patients believed that they were not the source of any problems inside the ward and that it was either other patients or staff who needed to be monitored. These patients were also keen to show that they had "nothing to hide". They linked camera use to wrongdoing inside the ward, and as they had done nothing wrong, they were not too disturbed by them.

> P4: *"I am quite pleased. I am a bit unusual like that because I have nothing to hide".*
>
> P5: *"I don't really think oh there's someone watching me. I just think oh there's a camera there. I know that someone can see me".*

Linked to this, some staff also believed that anyone objecting to being monitored by CCTV was doing so on the basis that they wanted to get up to no good. Therefore, any opposition to CCTV surveillance aroused suspicion.

> S6: *"Well I just feel that if you don't like CCTV then you're probably one of them people that's doing something wrong like, it don't bother me, I'm*

not doing anything, I'm not doing anything wrong so I don't mind being recorded or on CCTV".

S12: *"If you're not doing anything wrong, no need to worry about it. If you're doing something wrong, you need to worry about it but if you're doing nothing wrong don't worry about it".*

Mental capacity and camera awareness

The cameras' ability to discipline behaviour inside the ward is also linked to the deterrence of certain behaviours. For example, the impetus for the use of cameras in open street and shopping mall areas was linked to making these spaces safe by deterring crime (Clarke, 1997; Von Hirsh, 2002; Welsh and Farrington, 2007). Some patients also believed in the deterrence aspects of the cameras. A deterrence for these patients often related to petty crimes such as theft of their personal belongings or breaking ward rules such as establishing romantic relationships and liaisons with other patients. It also related to more serious crimes such as attacks on them.

P3: *"Where there are black-spots [blind-spots] it's obviously not going to be effective. But it does deter criminals and it is a way of bringing justice".*

P8: *"I mean like we're in the activity room now ... at the end of the day you don't want someone having too much fun and doing things that upset other people erm so CCTV is a good thing".*

Any deterrence of behaviour is dependent on the patient's capacity to understand this function of the cameras. Below, P8 describes how she had noticed the cameras even though when she arrived on the ward she was quite unwell.

P8: *"I'm not gonna lie I wasn't in a great state when I came in but you know I noticed the cameras".*

Several patients inside all three PICUs were aware that the ward had cameras inside it and believed the cameras were there to watch them. However, the mental health ward does not only care for those patients who have a mental health condition. There were also other patients inside the ward whose mental health condition was linked to other health factors such as learning disability or severe autism. The behaviour of these patients remained unchanged despite the presence of the cameras. During fieldwork observations, these patients continued to engage in behaviours that were risky and unsafe. For example, one woman continued to take her clothes off in all areas of the ward, including directly in front of a camera. Similarly, a male patient often ran uncontrollably through one ward and across the courtyard area despite being seen by staff. These patients were not affected or disturbed by cameras and neither did the cameras deter their behaviour.

Reason for the cameras

CCTV as evidence

In light of having no information about the cameras, both patients and staff surmised as to the reason for the cameras being inside the ward. Very few patients had any direct experience with the cameras. For instance, they had not been involved in any circumstance where an incident had been caught on camera in which they, another patient or staff had been implicated. Hence they, like staff, also tended to rely on wider political discourses to explain their presence in the ward. These included the idea that CCTV stops certain behaviours, such as patients attempting to commit suicide or stealing. That the cameras would provide clear evidence that would exonerate them when something went wrong in the ward, even though in one site the cameras did not record and in another site, the system was broken and unable to consistently record during most of the research period. That because the hospital is a public building, it would be a target for terrorism and that patients in mental hospitals are more likely to hurt each other, even though patients are more likely to attack staff than other patients (Noble and Rodgers, 1989).

> P3: *"I mean if there was an event and something happened like CCTV recording could be used as evidence".*
>
> P2: *"Ultimately the patient is being watched first and foremost. The management need evidence and need to provide evidence to the police and tribunal to show why I am here".*
>
> P4: *"I think from 1999 or about then anyway to 2001, three people killed themselves on x ward. I think they might have cameras to make sure that no one does that in here".*
>
> P5: *"Well you know that you're covered if something happens. You know that you're in control".*
>
> P7: *"Erm I automatically assumed that there was CCTV installed because it's a public building open to terrorism".*

Proof of innocence

Those few patients who did have some experience with cameras believed that the cameras were inside the ward to show their innocence when they have been attacked by other patients. For these and most other patients feeling safe inside the ward was a big factor in their recovery. Below, P14 describes an altercation with another patient in which he also implicates staff for not doing their job properly, especially in how they undertake the task of watching over him.

> P14: *"the second time err somebody [another patient] who kept on borrowing coke cola off me and wanting pound coins, and then it got to the point at the end of the day when I'd just had enough of that, lending him stuff. So I said, look here mate, that's enough of that let's get on in here enoughs, enough. He said don't shout at me. I said I'm not shouting at you, I'm not, and started to walk away. As I'm walking away, he came for me and lamped me in the back of the head. All on camera! Four members of staff around, so they all got to know but if it wasn't on camera, it'd be my word against his, and the witness's word [staff who were present] but witnesses aren't always reliable as you think because not everyone is watching … what they should be watching".*

Assuming patients are "up to no good"

Several patients, who were aware that the ward had cameras inside them, were angry and upset that they had not been given any information about them. They were unsure why the cameras were in the ward and how information about them was being used. As already stated in this chapter, this was not only contrary to data protection legislation and code of practice. It also led to some patients feeling that they were not valued and were not to be trusted. The lack of information about the purpose of the cameras also led to the feeling that the cameras were there to spy on them. These beliefs also increased anxiety for some patients, resulting in behaviours that were normal responses, but could be conceived as abnormal in the context of the mental health ward. Therefore, some patients viewed the cameras as a threat.

> P2: *"I was angry, why are we under surveillance? I was checking my bedroom, toilet, which would compromise my sanity".*
>
> P10: *"And, I'm a bit worried. I've got my injection tomorrow and I don't need it cos I'm not psychotic. I do worry about the cameras because I think they're recording our interview now … I sometimes think are they recording our speech, what we're talking about? I don't know. Do they do that?"*
>
> P11: *"No I think it's a breakdown of trust … because I think you need to have a good relationship between nurses, doctors and the patients and if you're monitoring people you don't, you suspect they're up to no good. You got to have some level, more level of trust and obviously, there has to be monitoring going on but it's more, you need the human connection and it [CCTV] dehumanises people. It dehumanises people and I think it's just, it's no good".*

These views expressed by patients raise several interconnected concerns. By not having enough information about how the cameras are used, all three patients have identified how this has adversely impacted their mental health. The main purpose of the hospital is to provide a safe space or asylum away from mainstream society. This aspect of being somewhere safe was undermined as some patients believed that there were more cameras in the ward than there were and that the cameras could do more than they did, such as record conversation. It is these aspects that have led to what P11 describes as a breakdown in trust because as P11 states the presence of the cameras start from the premise that they, as patients, are not trustworthy and are "*up to no good*". Molin et al. (2016) describe the importance of establishing trustful relationships with patients, where patients value the interaction they have with staff. For some patients, this relationship would always be difficult because the mere presence of the cameras suggested that they were not to be trusted. Therefore, any effort by staff to engage with patients also becomes undermined because the presence of the cameras for these patients suggests a conflicting relationship.

Accountability

Some patients also accepted the cameras because they realised that the cameras made staff accountable. Edal et al. (2019) describe how patients in their research felt powerless inside the ward. For example, through a sense of feeling worthless because the ward experience was ruled by not being allowed to do things, and by the infantilising of patients, or only seeing the person as their mental health diagnosis.

> P2: "*On a macro level management are also being watched. They could be held accountable*".
>
> P6: "*Case anything ever happens. Also, err if a patient's badly treated, they can play it back … it's all recording*".

Those patients who were also suspicious of staff motives did not just want the cameras to record visual footage but also sound.

> P4: "*I think if they have CCTV with sound it is a good thing. I think it would be very useful to stop members of staff misbehaving if there is litigation*".

Several patients also believed that the cameras might protect them from other patients. Loss of personal items was often linked with theft. Incidents inside the ward were often associated with patients not knowing where they had left their belongings and believing that other patients or staff had helped themselves to their personal items. Below, patients describe how other patients can compromise their safety inside the ward.

> P7: *"Yes, most certainly…it's a very good idea for the safety, security, protection … erm illegal entry into your…room and for the protection of your belongings".*
>
> P10: *"It makes sure that people aren't … stealing things".*
>
> *P3: "One of the patients was really staring at me. People [staff] say keep 10 feet away from him. If there's a camera it might be a deterrent. I don't know, it's not particularly nice for people to be under surveillance".*

Using cameras to research patients

One patient believed that the cameras might be used for research purposes. The idea that the body might be surveilled for research purposes inside the ward is not inconceivable. Henderson (1994: 935) draws on Foucault's power/knowledge coupling to suggest that "micro" practices of nursing are reliant upon the knowledge that is developed not only at a ward level but also at an individual level and that "the way the body is perceived and examined at this 'micro' level is instrumental to how knowledge is constituted".

> P12: *"Erm maybe they collect for research perhaps I don't know. I mean … I'm sure there is research that goes on here into mental health err you know statistics and whatnot, and maybe the CCTV maybe plays a role in that. Err I wouldn't, I don't understand how that would work … any way that they can collect data they will use I'm sure. I think so yeah".*

In the previous chapter, S2 describes how the ability to scrutinise a patient's behaviour when in seclusion allowed her to enhance her understanding of a patient's mental health condition: *"It lets us know what they're like cos everybody has their own, I like to think of it as a mask they put on when they come to the communal area so sort of hide who they are".* Foucault (cited in Gordon, 1980) believed that power appears in an array of micro-situations, and it is only by understanding internal controls which provide the patient with technologies of the self, that it becomes possible for them to construct themselves in accordance with the ruling power/knowledge configuration. Therefore, the "micro" practices operating within the hospital at the ward level, as well as at the individual patient level, are central to the development of knowledge.

It is through examining the body of the patient at this "micro" level in seclusion that S2 was able to create meaning, which then becomes instrumental in how knowledge about that patient is constructed. This unimpeded gaze by S2, according to Sewell and Barker (2007: 358), suggests that this form of surveillance will reveal the "essential truth" about the patient. They also go on to say suggest that what is also central to Foucault's ideas around power/knowledge is that the surveillance of the patient does not stop at revealing the truth; it also "*creates* truth". Therefore, S2 is not only interested in observing the patient, but the observation is also done with a purpose where she becomes involved in finding out which of the patient's behaviour are real and which are a mask or fake. In this way, the cameras do not only provide access to what was previously unseen behaviour. They also influence how staff view patient behaviour as they assist them in the unravelling of patient behaviour to identify what is real. Therefore, the cameras not only act as a learning tool, in doing so, they also construct a truth about the patient. The unobtrusive watching of patients is not limited to that particular patient. It is also applicable to other patients and in this way contributes to wider knowledge, based on understanding the behaviour of patients with a mental health condition.

Responses to CCTV surveillance

Bedroom cameras

Most patients inside site 3 knew that there were cameras inside their bedroom and that they had been told about them. A few patients stated that they had agreed to camera observation so that they could get undisturbed sleep during the night. However, the majority of patients, including those who had consented to their use, admitted that they did not like having a camera in their bedroom. A few staff were aware of this and confirmed that generally patients did not like bedroom cameras.

> S27: *"Most of them [patients] will insist on being moved to another ward where the cameras are not there you know, yeah ... most of them will not want the cameras in their room to be honest".*

Privacy in the context of the bedroom was perceived by patients as having the space inside the ward to be themselves and not to be judged by staff as having another motive for their behaviour, as explained by P12 below.

> P12: *"Yeah it's not nice err if I'm thinking sometimes, I like to pace. It's something I've done my whole life and I felt like I couldn't do that in my room because they might look at it and think oh you know, what's wrong with him. You know its stuff like that, you can't, like I can't feel like myself".*

For P12, either the lack of understanding as to how bedroom cameras were operated or that he did not believe that staff were not watching him all the time when he was in his bedroom resulted in a source of stress. It was the not knowing when and how he was being observed which resulted in him conforming his behaviour to what he believed staff expected from him. The panoptic aspect of the camera resulted in him having to choose between whether he continued to pace and have staff believe that there was something wrong with him, or stop pacing in his room and possibly become overwhelmed by his emotions. He, therefore, found himself in a difficult position as the consequence of not pacing could equally result in him looking troubled and further perpetuating that there was something wrong with him.

Discharge from the ward

The visibility of the cameras and the verifiability of staff watching the cameras meant that several patients believed that behaviour observed on camera footage would influence their discharge from the ward. These patients believed that CCTV evidence of their behaviour inside the ward was used to determine their recovery and eventual discharge from the ward. This was the case in all three PICUs even though in site 1 the cameras were live feeds only. For these patients, cameras were a way of showing the clinical team that they could control their behaviour around staff and other people.

> P2: *"It's a two-way conversation between me and management and the management and me. Basically, it's my way of saying I am ready to move away".*
>
> P5: *"Erm well the patients need constant monitoring because that's, that's why they've been brought here. Erm to sort of study their behaviour, understand what treatments need to be given".*
>
> P8: *"Erm I imagine it goes higher and higher up the hierarchy erm and then is analysed and people's behaviours is analysed you know letting them get release and stuff like that. Like err Dr x [names consultant psychiatrist] who is coming here. I'm sure he's reviewed all the CCTV and stuff to see how people are behaving ... To think that I know my doctors can err be seeing me. Hello (P8 laughs, looks and waves at the camera in the room) I'm being good. Please let me out!"*

For some patients, conformity was also linked to their belief that the cameras were a way of directly communicating with their consultant psychiatrist. Most patients did not see their consultant psychiatrist daily. The consultant psychiatrist's presence inside the ward was often associated with their absence from it. Inside all three PICUs, patients often met with their consultant once a week during multidisciplinary ward meetings, often referred to as the weekly ward round. Ethnographic fieldwork notes describe how patients were often more anxious and agitated on these days. The build-up to ward round day and the actual day appeared to be a tense time for patients. This was the day that they had the opportunity to directly influence their consultant psychiatrist through a face-to-face encounter with them. It was also the day that patients hoped that they may find out about a discharge date. During ward round days, there was also more than the usual number of staff inside the ward. This was partly associated with some staff being involved in ward round meetings and other staff in the management of patients who may not get the outcome that they might have hoped for such as discharge from the ward, resulting in them becoming distressed or angry.

This heightened level of activity, which also included a range of other people coming into the ward, such as a social worker, housing officer and other professional workers who were not regular visitors to the ward, sets these days apart from the everyday. Inside two research sites, the ward round took place inside rooms that were located in the ward, and any visitor entering the ward would be quickly ushered away by staff into the ward office or the meeting room. On these days, there was a sense of movement and change, and it was the potential for the patient's circumstances to change which made them agitated. Naik describes how ward rounds can also be intimidating experiences for staff:

> Every Sunday evening, for three years, my stomach would be in knots about the impending ward round. Speaking out loud in a team of more than 10 other professionals was daunting to say the least.
>
> (Naik, 2017)

The hierarchical nature of these meetings is located in the individualising power of the psychiatrist who also has to show that she or he is in charge of the patient, even when they are not always physically present inside the ward (Foucault, 2008). Relational power in the context of the ward round is therefore demonstrated in the psychiatrist's ability to be in control of the patient's care. Carey et al. (2015) reported that 48 per cent of patients in their research reported that they felt anxious and threatened at ward round meetings. The majority of patients inside all three research sites found the ward round meetings disempowering. These patients felt that they were not able to participate in these meetings and believed that they were spoken to, rather than heard (O'Driscoll et al., 2014). During fieldwork observations, a few patients also believed that the ward rounds were a waste of time as the only reason they believed they had to continue to stay inside the ward was that they did not have anywhere else to go as they were homeless. Therefore, ward rounds became a source of tension for patients for several reasons including the inability to influence their consultant psychiatrist that they were ready to be discharged, which resulted in their stress. In these circumstances, although patients were not wholly sure whether their consultant psychiatrist viewed camera footage or not, the possibility that they could, or would be able to, was a source of reassurance as well as a source of stress.

Hidden cameras

Surveillance in shaping people's behaviour is based on knowing that they are looked at, or being surveilled (Lyon, 2002; Marx, 2009). The intensive nature of surveillance in the ward demonstrated through a range of techniques, such as nurse observations, staff stationed in various communal areas of the ward, ward information leaflets telling patients they are in the ward to be observed, the openness of the ward office which enabled staff to see out into communal areas, the visibility of CCTV cameras and CCTV monitors, all constituted part of an assemblage of techniques inside the ward to let patients know that they were always being monitored. This intensity of monitoring led several patients to believe in the possibility of hidden cameras inside the ward. This belief that there may be hidden cameras in the ward provided a source of psychological stress for several patients, and it also influenced their behaviour to the point that it distorted how they attempted to shape their behaviour, especially in their efforts to show others that their mental health was improving.

Latané (1981: 343) describes social impact as about any change in "psychological states and subjective feelings, motives and emotions, cognitions and beliefs, values and behaviour, that occur in an individual, human, or animal, as a result of the real, implied or imagined presence or actions of other individuals". His theoretical analysis suggests that even the imagined presence of others can have an impact on patient and staff behaviour. During fieldwork observations, staff tended to congregate in certain parts of the ward when they wanted relief from patients, the cameras, and certain peers and managers. Inside two research sites, this area tended to be the kitchen linked to the patient dining room. Patients could not see staff in there because the hatch from the kitchen to the dining room was often closed and locked when not in use. Staff tended to congregate here, rather than use the dedicated staff room, which was separate from the ward office because technically they were still inside the ward working and not on a break. There were no cameras inside these spaces, and staff could have a reason for being there, for example, they were counting cutlery or making hot drinks for patients. For patients, there were very few places like these where they could go and be themselves. In all three research sites, staff believed that the patient bedroom was where patients could retreat if they found the ward environment stressful. However, the visibility of the real cameras and their continuous observation led some patients to believe that the ward had hidden cameras inside it, especially in their bedroom.

> S6: *"you do talk to them [patients] sometimes and they say erm like they're recording me in my bedroom and like, no there ain't no cameras in your bedroom".*
>
> S10: *"like Big Brother type thing but you try and tell em [patients] no we don't put cameras in your bedroom, you know what I mean, that's your area*

you can go and do what you want in that area. I don't particularly want to see it on a monitor in the office".

P11: *"Well, there's the obvious ones and there's also hidden cameras".*

A few staff linked patient belief of hidden cameras to their mental health condition, especially where they believed that the cameras had a negative impact on the patient's mental health condition.

S7: *"Like a lot of patients, when they're very poorly believe they're being recorded and things are being wire-tapped and so on. A lot of it does feed into delusions and we have had that, even though we've only got a small amount of cameras".*

Despite being told by staff that there were no hidden cameras inside spaces such as bedrooms, bathrooms and toilets, patients tended to believe that these spaces had cameras inside them.

P2: *"I had to enquire if that dome shape in my room [P2 is referring to a dome-shape mirror] was CCTV and they told me it wasn't. I asked about the long-shaped box in the bathroom. I thought it was a microphone. They told me it wasn't".*

P3: *"someone said to me, a patient, the cameras are so small you can't see them. I think it was some babble from a paranoid patient. Maybe there are tiny cameras, I don't know, but I can't imagine".*

Patients who believed that the ward had hidden cameras inside it also believed that camera footage was observed wider than the immediate staff group.

S27: *"The patient was just anti-camera and he will think the camera is government, so he will be talking to the camera about sections, appeal, why he's being held in here".*

P2: *"It's a two-way conversation between me and the management and the management and me. Basically, it's my way of saying I am ready to move away".*

Most patients who believed that camera footage was viewed widely also believed that any footage would also be viewed by their consultant psychiatrist.

P8: *"It's just interesting, isn't it? To think that I know my doctors can err be seeing me. Hello (she laughs and waves to the camera again) (Both laugh). I'm being good. Please let me out! (She talks directly to the camera) (Both laugh). I'm not going crazy. Don't worry I'm not offending this nice lady (she laughs). Yeah, no, no, it's a, it's to view interaction, isn't it?"*

As someone who is in charge of their care, most patients were not sure how their consultant psychiatrist knew when they were well enough to leave the ward as they were mostly absent from it. Maintaining control over their behaviour and being compliant was therefore not limited to those areas of the ward where the cameras were visible. The narratives described above of suspicion and the belief that people in authority, whether that is managers, their consultant psychiatrist or even people beyond the ward such as government officials who were involved in observing them, was simultaneously a source of reassurance and a source of stress for these patients. Patient behaviour was not limited to influencing staff; it was extended to people beyond the ward that they could not easily access and whom they believed could influence their discharge from the ward. For some patients, the need to influence their consultant psychiatrist, hospital managers and mental health tribunal members was more important than influencing staff. For these patients, the idea of hidden cameras was more problematic as they attempted to discipline their own behaviour when they were alone inside their bedroom. Their actions in resisting hidden camera surveillance did not always result in pro-social behaviour. While these patients believed that being seen may result in the approval of their consultant psychiatrist, for example, P8 (cited above) who believed that her consultant psychiatrist might be looking at her interacting with me during the interview and hoping that she was making a good impression on him. Although P8 gained some reassurance that this pro-social behaviour might earn her some credibility with her consultant psychiatrist, her attempt (see below) to gain relief from what she believed was constant observation resulted in covering up what she thought were hidden cameras inside her bedroom. These actions (as expanded in the next section), at times, seriously disrupted the ward environment.

P8: *"I don't think there's any in patient rooms are there? (I: No). So, I mean I did see a little, a little black box like that (P8 points to what looks like an old smoke alarm system which has been covered up on the ceiling of the activity room) with a small hole in it and when I first arrived I did cover it up with toothpaste, just in case ... Just cos you know, you want a degree of privacy".*

When staff described patient concerns about the cameras, they often used clinical terms, which they linked to the patient's mental health condition. Therefore, responses by patients to cameras, whether these were linked to real or imagined cameras, have the potential to be documented in their patient record in a negative and symptomatic way. The cameras, again whether real or imagined, also create stress for patients at a time when they are not fully in control of their behaviour.

> S2: *"We have a couple of people who are very paranoid and if there's a camera we are recording them, and we'll be watching them and like making fun of them and stuff like that".*
>
> S15: *"It causes patients quite a lot of paranoia erm ... because they're being watched so when you've got paranoid patient the fact that they are being watched only fuels their paranoia".*
>
> S16: *"where you have acutely unwell erm often psychotic very often paranoid individuals and they're at a point that it's acute crisis really err it's often reference to me, who's watching me, is it the government?"*
>
> S19: *"Just patients may be getting paranoid about them sometimes, but you know especially in the communal areas they haven't got a choice whether they're on CCTV or not".*
>
> S21: *"Some patients can be paranoid that you're constantly watching them through the camera or feel like you could have the screen up in the office watching so that could be an issue for some patients if they feel that, you know, you're, they're constantly being watched in their bedroom".*
>
> S24: *"Some people [patients] prefer them but some people because of the red light here, cos most of our patients, a high degree of them are paranoid schizophrenic so the idea of someone watching them on camera does not sit well with them".*

Resisting camera surveillance

Away from CCTV cameras, Boyne (2000: 295) suggests that there are many examples of the failure of the panoptical paradigm inside asylums. He cites Goffman and states that within the asylum, there are many examples of resistance and "strategies of subversion". For example, Goffman (1961) describes how space was used inside the ward by patients as a means of disrupting the totalising effect of the asylum. First, "there was space that was off-limits or out of bounds". Second, "there was *surveillance space*, the area a patient needed no special excuse for being in", and third, there was "space ruled by less than usual staff authority", which Goffman referred to as "free places" (Goffman, 1961: 203–204). It was not just out of bound spaces or free places that patients could go to in order to resist surveillance. They could also disrupt surveillance by being inside surveillance spaces, by using these spaces to show staff that they could control their behaviour. During fieldwork observations, several patients used communal areas of the ward so that they could demonstrate to staff that they were ready to leave the ward. For some patients, being inside these surveillance spaces or communal areas of the ward required a lot of effort. For example, some patients did not want to be seen by staff because they could recall how they were when they first came into the ward. Other patients did not want to use communal areas of the ward because they did not like or trust certain staff and did not enjoy being in their company, or because they had always lived on their own and found the company of others stressful. Therefore, being inside communal spaces was difficult for some patients who knew that they had to perform within this space to show staff that they were able to master their behaviour and in turn demonstrate their readiness to leave the ward. Yar's (2003: 264) suggestion that patients are not "passive objects of a normalising gaze (on the way to becoming 'docile')" is demonstrated in this and other situations where patients managed their visibility.

While patients were less reluctant to talk about the different ways in which they attempted to resist surveillance or manage their visibility, staff gave several examples of how patients attempted to minimise or reduce the effects of surveillance. Except for one PICU where patients had managed to burn part of a CCTV camera inside the courtyard area, by removing the camera lens and burning the plastic lens with a cigarette, most actions were generally individual responses and not always carried out effectively. Most of this section draws on some of Marx's (2003) surveillance neutralisation techniques adopted by patients when attempting to resist CCTV surveillance.

Distorting moves

Marx (2003) describes distorting moves as actions by which people manipulate surveillance processes in such ways that the data becomes disrupted. Those patients who understood the nature of CCTV surveillance were able to manipulate cameras better and therefore were able to control how they were seen. For example, P14, who was pro-CCTV cameras, did not mind them and changed his behaviour accordingly.

> P14: *"The disadvantages were privacy and the fact that you don't act the same as what you would do when you're on camera".*

P14 understood how CCTV surveillance functioned and could weigh-up how to use such surveillance to his advantage. He believed that he was able to make the cameras work for him because he knew how to manipulate and distort surveillance by discovering whether the cameras were fake or real.

> P14: *"so situations like is that camera really a camera or is it a dummy camera? If it's a dummy camera I'd just act like my normal self, if it's a real camera then I have to put on a, on a front and pretend to be somebody I'm not".*

Similarly, P8 was also someone who did not mind the cameras in the ward. P8 often played up to the cameras, for example, by gesticulating in a friendly way at them. She often held her fingers up in a V-sign (which she referred to as her "rock-on" sign) or waved at cameras in the communal areas. P8 did this throughout our interview which was in a room that had a camera inside it. I also observed her doing the same inside the ward. She treated the cameras, especially those in the communal area and courtyard, as if they were real "people" watching her as opposed to some faceless technology that was just recording her:

> P8: *"I give them my rock-on sign. (I: I notice you doing that now). Yeah, I like I don't know, I just like, they're watching me, like, I'm still here. I'm still remembering who I am but I'm not going to turn it around and be offensive erm but I am still me".*

While P14 distorted the information that staff might have about him through the process of demonstrating conformity and showing that he could control his behaviour. P8's distortion of surveillance was linked to her desire to be recognised as an individual. P8 did not see herself as communicating with the cameras but with those staff that she believed were watching her through the camera. P8 distorted surveillance by treating the camera as if it were a person and not a piece of equipment. This was different from performing for the cameras (described in more detail in the next section). P8 interacted with the cameras in ways that showed that she would not be ignored by staff and she attempted to do this in a playful way.

To some extent, P1 (see Field note 011 below), in our interview, also described how he attempted to maintain his personhood and individuality in the context of surviving seclusion. Again, he did not respond to his surveillance negatively and attempted to maintain his dignity and autonomy by being cooperative but also trying to remember that he was also a person. The field note is an interview with P1 (not audio-taped) in which I also gave him a written account of our interview at his request. The quotes are from this written account.

> Field note 011: *"You told me when you were 'in the blocks' [seclusion] you decided to 'embrace your power'. You said, 'they put music on, so I started dancing', and that this made you feel better. You told me you enjoyed 'dancing around'. You said you had your 'boxers on' and that you were 'dancing like a stripper...to give them* [*meaning staff*] *a show'. You thought the best way to embrace your power was to 'enjoy yourself', while you were in seclusion".*

These distorting moves were different from simply performing for the cameras. These patients recognised that CCTV technology could not only expose their body but that their behaviour would be judged by staff who could see them. The need to know whether the cameras are fake or not and the desire to interact in certain ways with the cameras (for example, playfully) was driven by their need to let those doing CCTV surveillance know that they were not negatively influenced by such monitoring.

Performing for the cameras

Some patients accepted the cameras because they enjoyed the possibility of being watched by other people and performing in front of them. Patients who enjoyed performing in front of the cameras did not necessarily do this to distort surveillance. They just enjoyed the fact that they were being looked at. For some patients, being looked at was not limited to staff inside the ward. They also believed that an audience beyond the ward may also be watching them. This was particularly the case inside one PICU where a camera was located next to the television set directly opposite a seating area where patients sat to watch the television. This prompted some patients to believe that CCTV footage may be recorded for popular television programmes like Gogglebox, where the public watch ordinary people watching a television programme and their reactions to the programme, or the television programme Big Brother, where the public watch participants engaged in daily living activities locked in a house, with no contact with the outside world. The latter programme is not dissimilar to their own experience of being locked up inside the ward with very little contact with the outside world.

> Field note 130: *"I ask her if she has noticed that the ward has cameras. She tells me she has noticed one by the tv [television]. I ask her what she thinks about it. She tells me she that likes it. She asks me if I'm recording for my research. I tell her no. She says it's a shame, she wants to be on tv and that this is what she's wanted all her life".*
>
> P3: *"Yeah one of my favourite tv shows is Celebrity Big Brother at the end of the day erm, I always ... wanted to go on Big Brother".*
>
> P8: *"and other things as well people [other patients] act up for the cameras. They act like they're bloomin Madonna or something ...".*
>
> P14: *"I do a lot of dancing when I'm outside and I'm on camera from multiple angles ... and I thought to myself do you know what I'm doing some really good [moves] and I wouldn't mind some camera footage ... I was quite impressed with my own moves I wouldn't mind some of the footage and then play it back to music and make an art piece out of it because it's, it's been recorded isn't it ... But they won't give me the footage. I did ask politely as well".*

Mathiesen (1997: 223) has argued that panopticism and synopticism have developed in fusion with each other. This fusion, according to him, is evident in Orwell's (1949) "*Nineteen Eighty-Four*" novel where panopticism and synopticism completely merge "through a screen in your living room you saw

Big Brother, just as Big Brother saw you". Mathiesen (1997: 226) suggests that within synoptic space, celebrities are seen as important figures who, through their visibility, "actively filter and shape information". Inside mental health wards where patients become depersonalised and have little say in who they are, celebrity status can for some patients take on greater importance. Also, Koskela suggests that surveillance is not always perceived as "restricting and repressive" and that people "*play with* various forms of surveillance equipment". Her analysis of surveillance in this way suggests that patients are often "weary of being passive targets" of surveillance. She further suggests that most "performances that people engage in are not necessarily their own creation, but often mimic assorted 'commercial idols' presented in reality TV shows such as Big Brother, where imitating surveillance is a key part of the appeal of such shows" (Koskela, 2012: 54).

While some staff were aware that patients liked to perform for the cameras, other staff tended to link patient's camera performances to their mental disorder (usually personality disorders) and as a form of attention-seeking behaviour.

> S8: *"I mean knowing that they're on camera they might behave in a different way, I mean particularly service users [patients] with personality disorders. They will display certain behaviours to gain attention and they know that you're watching them on camera, and I've seen that a few times, yeah".*

Sexualised performances

The previous two chapters have highlighted concerns around the gendered nature of surveillance. Managers, for example (see Chapter 3), believed that CCTV surveillance had the potential to deter male patients from entering female ward areas, while Chapter 4 highlights how bedroom cameras provided staff with the opportunity to look at patient's sexualised behaviours. Patients who performed intimate and sexualised behaviours did not always do so in a deliberate and controlled way, where they had control over their behaviour. For example, Koskela (2012: 55) describes how in the move from "voyeurism to exhibition", "camgirls" and "camguys" used "camming" to perform live online self-presentations, where they turn their real-life images into "reality porn", to gain some control of what and how these images are presented.

A few staff described how some patients engaged in intimate performance activities such as masturbating inside their bedroom which stopped them from using the cameras. Patients knew when the cameras were operational as a red light lit up inside their bedroom when the camera was switched on, or in seclusion where there was no respite from being watched. Below, staff describe the different ways in which patients, both male and female, change the nature of surveillance by engaging in sexualised behaviour or by exposing their body either in their bedroom or in seclusion.

> S27: *"but the girls are so bad, men are better yeah, men do it also, lie on their bed make sure the camera is looking at them … They put the light on. So, women in x [names another ward which uses CCTV in bedrooms] will do that almost every day so you're forced to shut up the screen".*
>
> S3: *"or they can get naked and stuff".*
>
> S8: *"Or take their clothes off and go Look at Me!"*

Inside mental health wards, these behaviours are often linked to the patient's mental health condition. For example, Bowers et al. (2014) reported that most incidents of exposure of the naked body and public masturbation happened in the first two weeks of admission. While these actions might close down camera surveillance, they are not done deliberately and consciously by those patients who engage in these intimate acts. The majority of these patients cannot control this behaviour, and it is their inability to control this behaviour, which makes them vulnerable in the context of the ward. Koskela (2012: 55) also states that "we should not lose sight of the fact that most instances of surveillance remain oppressive or simply sustains unequal power". Therefore, although this behaviour had some success in that it sometimes closed down surveillance, it raised other concerns about patient safety inside the ward. This was particularly problematic when the patient was engaging in sexualised behaviour inside the seclusion room. S5 (below) describes how this behaviour has a wider audience.

> S5: *"They are observed by one person but when you are on the camera it is more than that. You might think you are only observed by that particular person who is allocated to supervise you in seclusion. It could be that those pictures are seen by many people that you don't trust especially".*

Patient performance in front of cameras distorted their surveillance in several ways. The desire to be on a television programme or be seen on the internet meant that some patients purposefully acted out in front of the cameras. These patients often performed what they believed were dance moves that would get them noticed by people beyond the ward. This behaviour was influenced by the visibility of the cameras and the cameras' ability to capture them from a range of angles. While these constitute playful responses in which patients fantasise about a different life, those responses where they expose their naked body or participate in sexualised behaviours in front of the cameras has the potential for more sinister outcomes.

Blocking cameras

Marx (2003: 379) describes blocking and masking moves as explicit forms of intervention that are undertaken by surveillant subjects to physically block "access to communication or to render it ... unusable". The staff gave several examples of how patients attempted to block the camera view. These attempts were not only on cameras located in the communal and courtyard areas of the ward, but they also included the camera in seclusion and the camera located inside the patient bedroom.

> S2: *"They've [patients] tried to cover up the camera in the seclusion room. Like we've had to go to clean up ketchup and sandwiches and stuff like that off em cos they will try and cover that up and they'll try and cover up the observation or the observation window so you can't see them".*
>
> S1: *"The most common thing is food, smearing food on em".*
>
> S11: *"One by the tv, that one gets covered up".*
>
> S15: *"Or people [patients] put toothpaste a lot on them ... or paper, cover them or things like that".*
>
> S27: *"They [patients] normally cover them, so if they don't like it in their room some of them climb up there and cover them ... They know they are lenses they cover them".*

Patients also described how they put toothpaste, shaving foam, hand cream and other items on mirrors and smoke alarms in their bedroom because they believed that these were hidden cameras inside their rooms. Hence, blocking moves were not only deployed on real cameras but also on those cameras that patients believed were hidden. Blocking moves were also problematic where the patient believed they were targeting hidden cameras. The act of attempting to damage hidden cameras inside the ward which included fire alarms, water sprinklers and various other safety features meant that occasionally patients also managed to break these features. This sometimes resulted in the locking down of the ward, where patients were often confined to their bedroom until the safety feature had been fixed or the fire service gave permission for ward activities to resume.

Breaking moves

Alongside attempting to block camera view, some patients also attempted to break or damage cameras. Marx (2003: 381) describes breaking moves as the "crudest form of neutralisation". In the first two quotes (below), S1 and S7 describe how patients placed in seclusion have damaged the camera. However, rather than questioning whether it was the correct decision to use a CCTV camera in seclusion, S7 describes how the camera was changed for a different model which was harder to destroy. The rhizomatic nature of surveillance and its ability to regenerate (see Haggerty and Ericson, 2000), that is when one system fails and another is deployed to take over, was demonstrated in how surveillance practices in seclusion are never questioned. Instead, new technologies are sought to resolve problems.

> S1: *"I mean there was the one lad [patient] that did manage to erm actually pull one. Yeah, they're high up but he managed to pull. He managed to get like a, we've got like a big block on the side and he climbed on that".*
>
> S7: *"It's mainly been like in seclusion when people [patients] have been poorly and like they've just been delusional and wanting to basically attack anything and don't like the fact that there's a camera in there and can see them".*
>
> S7: *"and we had to have them taken down and different camera put in with a plate over it so it was like flat and you can't grab it, whereas before you could grab it".*

Some breaking moves were not feeble attempts at damaging the cameras and neither were they individualised responses. For example, S10 (below) describes how a patient managed to damage a camera in the courtyard area, and S11 describes how the camera in the female communal area was damaged. To cause this damage, these patients did not work alone.

> S10: *"The one outside, one of em [patient] actually took it off, put his cigarette on the lens to burn the lens so you couldn't see much".*
>
> S11: *"down the female pod as well that one's been hanging off … I think they just smashed it!"*

To block staff looking at them in their bedroom, staff also reported the different ways in which patients attempted to damage bedroom cameras on site 3.

> S24: *"Yeah, yeah, yeah so you can't see. Like scratching and he [patient] smeared stuff so you can't see through … but he was scratching, the view was fuzzy you can't really see".*
>
> S27: *"They will be fighting the camera trying to kick them out and you know once they have removed them, they can do silly things".*

Avoidance moves

Marx (2003) states that avoidance moves are passive and involve withdrawal from surveillance. Both staff and some patients identified those areas inside the ward and unit that they could go to when they wanted to get away from the cameras.

> S2: "*Cos there are places where you are not being observed on a camera, like the staff room or the actual communal area*".
>
> P8: "*Go in my room. Go in the bathroom ... there were previously blind spots, but I think they've covered them a lot more now cos I've been watching them put up, well I've been talking to them, electrician*". *[P8 is talking about the addition of new cameras inside one of the research site wards].*
>
> P9: "*Go to my bedroom. I assume there's no cameras there, is there?*"
>
> P12: "*I know a spot where I think there aren't any so I can sit there if I want to, not be, you know looked at by a camera*".

Although the majority of staff understood that there were no hidden cameras inside the ward, most patients continued to believe that the ward and privates spaces, including their bedrooms, did have hidden cameras located inside them.

Conclusion

In this chapter, I have outlined how their awareness, knowledge and emotional responses to cameras have impacted patients as subjects of camera surveillance inside the ward. The belief that there were hidden cameras inside their bedrooms and that their consultant psychiatrist may be watching live footage or recorded material from real and imagined cameras simultaneously created stress and reassurance for some patients. However, it was not the continuous observation that created their stress. It was the not knowing whether it was their consultant psychiatrist who was watching live feeds or recorded information that was problematic. Theoretical analysis of this implication is discussed in more detail in the next chapter.

The main practice implications arising out of this chapter identify that:

- Patients are not told about the cameras and that this is contrary to the Information Commissioner's Office Code of Practice for Surveillance Cameras (2017: 37).
- Patients and staff did not believe that they could do anything about the cameras, including complaining about them, even though some staff and patients felt uncomfortable with the cameras inside the ward.
- The presence of the cameras inside the ward perpetuates the belief that PICU patients are violent and aggressive.
- Camera placement inside patient bedrooms raises a safeguarding concern, especially for women patients.
- Camera placement in communal areas of the ward and inside their bedrooms restricted spaces where patients could go to get away from

being under observation. This affected patient's mental health and caused them to feel stressed.

- The presence of real cameras led some patients to believe that the ward also had hidden cameras. This also created stress and was not conducive to a therapeutic ward environment.
- Patients were not always passive about CCTV surveillance and adopted several strategies to undermine surveillance inside the ward.

Bibliography

Ball, K. (2009). "Exposure: Exploring the subject of surveillance," *Information, Communication and Society,* 12(2): 639–657.

Bowers, L. (2014). "Safewards: A new model of conflict and containment on psychiatric wards," *Journal of Psychiatric and Mental Health Nursing*, 21(6): 499–508.

Boyne, R. (2000). "Post-panopticism," *Economy and Society*, 29(2): 285–307.

Carey, C., Lally, J. and Abba-Aji, A. (2015). "Are psychiatric team meetings patient centered? A cross-sectional survey on patient views regarding multi-disciplinary team meetings," *Irish Journal of Psychological Medicine*, 32(2): 177–185.

Clarke, R.V. (1997). "Introduction", in R.V. Clarke (ed), *Situational Crime Prevention: Successful Case Studies*, 2nd Edition, New York: Harrow and Heston Publishers, pp. 1–42.

Edal, K., Natvik, E., Veseth, M., Davidson, L., Skjolberg, A., Dorte, G. and Moltu, C. (2019). "Being recognised as a whole person: A qualitative study of inpatient experience in mental health," *Issues in Mental Health Nursing*, 40(2): 88–96.

Ellis, D., Tucker, I. and Harper, D. (2013). "The affective atmospheres of surveillance," *Theory and Psychology*, 23(6): 716–731.

Elmer, G. (2012). "Panopticon – discipline – control," in K. Ball, K.D. Haggerty and D. Lyon (eds), *Routledge Handbook of Surveillance Studies*. London: Routledge, pp. 21–29.

Foucault, M. (1979). *Discipline and Punish: The Birth of the Prison*, New York: Vintage.

Foucault, M. (2008). *Psychiatric Power: Lectures at the Collège de France 1973–1974*, edited by Jacques Lagrange and translated by Graham Burchell, Basingstoke: Palgrave.

Goffman, E. (1961). *Asylums: Essays on the Social Situation of Mental Patients and Other Inmates*, New York: Anchor Books.

Gordon, C. (ed) (1980). *Michel Foucault Power/Knowledge: Selected Interviews and Other Writings 1972–1977 by Michel Foucault*, London: Harvester Wheatsheaf.

Haggerty, K.D. and Ericson, R.V. (2000). "The surveillant assemblage," *British Journal of Sociology*, 51(4): 605–622.

Haggerty, K.D. and Ericson, R.V. (eds) (2007). *The New Politics Surveillance and Visibility*, Toronto, Buffalo, London: University of Toronto Press.

Henderson, A. (1994). "Power and knowledge in nursing practice: the contribution of Foucault," *JAN Leading Global Nursing Research*, 20(5): 935–939.

Information Commissioner's Office. (2017). *In the Picture: A Data Protection Code of Practice for Surveillance Cameras and Personal Information*, Version 1.2 20170609. Available online: www2.le.ac.uk/offices/estates/documents/design-guides/cctv-code-of-practice.pdf [accessed 23 January 2021].

Koskela, H. (2000). "The gaze without eyes: Video-surveillance and the changing nature of urban space," *Progress in Human Geography*, 24(2): 243–265.

Koskela, H. (2012). "'You shouldn't wear that body': The problematic of surveillance and gender," in K. Ball, K.D. Haggerty and D. Lyon (eds), *Routledge Handbook of Surveillance Studies.* London: Routledge, pp. 49–56.

Latané, B. (1981). "The psychology of social impact," *American Psychology*, 36: 343–356.

Lyon, D. (2002). "Everyday surveillance: Personal data and social classifications," *Information, Communication and Society*, 5(2): 242–257.

Lyon, D. (2007). *Surveillance Studies: An Overview*, Cambridge: Polity Press.

Marx, G.T. (2003). "A tack in the shoe: Neutralising and resisting new surveillance," *Journal of Social Issues*, 59(2): 369–390.

Marx, G.T. (2009). "A tack in the shoe and taking off the shoe: Neutralisation and counter-neutralisation," *Surveillance and Society*, 6(3): 294–306.

Mathiesen, T. (1997). "The viewer society: Michel Foucault's 'Panopticon' revisited," *Theoretical Criminology*, 1(2): 215–233.

Molin, J., Graneheim, U.H. and Lindgren, B.-H. (2016). "Quality of interactions influences everyday life in psychiatric inpatient care – Patient's perspectives," *International Journal of Qualitative Studies on Health and Well-being*, 11: 1. Available online: https://doi.org/10.3402/qhw.vll.2987 [accessed 28 January 2021].

Naik, J. (2017). "How to survive a multidisciplinary team meeting," *Community Care*, 2 May 2017. Available online: www.communitycare.co.uk/2017/05/02/survive-multidisciplinary-team-meeting/ [accessed 28 January 2021].

Noble, P. and Rodgers, S. (1989). "Violence by psychiatric in-patients," *British Journal of Psychiatry,* 155(3): 384–390.

O'Driscoll, W., Livingstone, G., Lanceley, A., Nic a Bhaird, C., Xanthopoulou, P., Manonmani, I.W. and Raine, M.R. (2014). "Patient experience of MDT care and decision-making," *Mental Health Review Journal*, 19: 4–23.

Orwell, G. (1949). *Nineteen Eighty-Four*, London: Secker and Warburg.

Sewell, G. (2012). "Organisation, employees and surveillance," in K. Ball, K.D. Haggerty and D. Lyon (eds), *Routledge Handbook of Surveillance Studies*, London: Routledge, pp. 303–312.

Sewell, G. and Barker, J.R. (2007). "Neither good, nor bad, but dangerous: Surveillance as an ethical paradox," In S. Heir and J. Greenburg (eds), The Surveillance Studies Reader. Maidenhead: McGraw-Hill Education, Open University Press, pp. 354–367.

Solove, D.J. (2007). "I've got nothing to hide and other misunderstandings of privacy," *San Diego Law Review,* 44: 745–772.

Taylor, D. (ed) (2014). *Michel Foucault: Key Concepts*, London: Routledge.

Von Hirsch, A. (2002). "The ethics of public television surveillance," in A. Von Hirsch, D. Garland and A. Wakefield (eds), *Ethical and Social Perspectives on Situational Crime Prevention*, Oxford: Hart Publishing, pp. 59–76.

Welsh, B.C. and Farrington, D.P. (2007). *Closed-Circuit Television Surveillance and Crime Prevention*, Stockholm: Swedish National Council for Crime Prevention.

Webster, W.R. and Murakami Wood, D. (2009). "Living in surveillance societies: The normalization of surveillance in Europe and the threat of Britain's bad example," *Journal of Contemporary European Research*, 5: 259–273.

Yar, M. (2003). "Panoptic power and the pathologisation of vision: Critical reflections on the Foucauldian thesis," *Surveillance and Society*, 1(3): 254–271.

Chapter 6

Conclusion

The politics of surveillance and mental health

Introduction

This chapter is divided into two parts. The first part explores how undertaking research inside mental health wards has contributed to the current theoretical debate in the social understanding of CCTV cameras. The second part examines the use of CCTV cameras inside mental health wards and practice implications of this on the patient experience. Several themes already raised in previous chapters are consolidated in this chapter. These include the influence of sovereign power, panoptic power and pastoral power in the disciplining of patient behaviour inside the mental health ward, the criminalisation of patient's violent behaviour, the exposure of women's bodies in the creation of gender inequalities inside the ward and the undermining of ethical mental health practice as a result of increasing reliance on camera technology to monitor patients.

Sociological understanding of CCTV technology

Background

This research has drawn on Foucault's analysis of sovereign power, panoptic power and pastoral power as a framework to understand how practices inside the mental health ward are used to influence patient behaviour and conduct. To understand the empirical data and how CCTV cameras influence patient and staff behaviour, the research has also drawn on other theories and concepts within the different chapters. For example, empirical data in Chapters 3, 4 and 5 has shown that the cameras are not a "black box", passively passing information from one place to another. That the information that is captured by the cameras, whether that is from live feeds or recorded information, influences the nature of what is watched and seen (Bijker et al, 2012). Chapter 4 highlights how Levinas (2006) and Ellul's (1964) theorisation influences what is watched and seen and how the cameras become embedded in day-to-day practices inside the ward. Similarly, Marx's (1988) analysis of surveillance creep draws attention to how the cameras' initial application, for

DOI: 10.4324/9781003179306-6

example, as a means to open up difficult-to-supervise areas inside the ward (or blind-spots), are taken over by other agendas. For instance, the desire by staff to expand cameras from blind-spots inside the ward to those areas where there is likely to be more aggression and violent behaviour (or hot-spots) (see Chapters 4 and 5 for more detail). Although this research has also shown the rise of camera use inside mental health wards (see Chapter 4), it still remains the case that there is no national policy or local policy on how cameras should be used. Any advice on camera use is largely influenced by their experimental uses inside the ward of which some are then retrospectively incorporated into guidance documents (see Chapter 4).

The empirical data for this research builds upon Foucault's original analysis of sovereign power, panoptic power and pastoral power in the governance of patients inside the mental health ward. This analysis has been missing in mental health literature. Also, surveillance literature has underplayed the influence of individualised power embodied in authority figures, for example, the consultant psychiatrist. This research has shown the importance of the panoptic impact of the consultant psychiatrist, who, although largely invisible inside the ward, continued to influence the patient's behaviour through their absence. Foucault's (2009) analysis of pastoral power identifies three key features related to the positioning of the consultant psychiatrist inside the ward. These include the focus on the patient (the flock) and not the ward, the well-being of the patient and the individualising power of the psychiatrist in promoting the well-being of the patient. Foucault's analysis centred on aspects such as leadership skills in the context of the consultant psychiatrist's individualising power, where he does not directly link this aspect of pastoral power with panoptic power (Foucault, 2009). This research suggests that inside the mental health ward, the consultant psychiatrist held sovereign power in their ability to discharge the patient from the ward. They held pastoral power in their therapeutic relationship with the patient, and they held panoptic power in their continued presence and unavailability or invisibility inside the ward environment. Although they were largely absent from the ward, the consultant psychiatrist still knew how each patient was progressing in relation to their recovery. It was their knowledge about each patient which made the patient body visible inside the ward. Their ability to know how well the patient's recovery is progressing and at the same time not be seen inside the ward made it difficult for patients on two counts. First, it made it difficult for patients to influence them in their decision to discharge them from the hospital. Second, the patient was not always sure as to what was known about them by their consultant psychiatrist because they could not directly influence them.

Panopticism

Although Foucault (2008) believed that the mental health hospital was a "panoptic machine", there is surprisingly little research examining what he meant by this in the context of asylums and post-institutional mental health hospitals. Also, as Simon (2005) has noted, Foucault's analysis of the Panopticon has been both extensively criticised by numerous authors and analysed differently by others. Surveillance literature has also been criticised for focusing too heavily on the control aspect in the monitoring of people's behaviour, where authors such as Moore (2011) and Lyon (2001) have been critical about the lack of pastoral and productive aspect of surveillance practices. Lyon (2001: 3), for example, has theorised about the "Janus-faced" nature of surveillance, meaning that surveillance practices can often be simultaneously experienced as caring and controlling. The empirical data for this research suggests that surveillance practices feature heavily inside mental health wards. The mental health ward is different because surveillance practices are not just about influencing or changing behaviour. The success of the ward lies in its ability to cure the patient, where Foucault (2008) also described the mental health hospital as a "curing machine".

Modern mental health hospitals, like asylums, are also reliant on practices that are more akin to sovereign power. For example, locked wards, the use of seclusion practices, forced medication and full-body restraint of patients are some of the ways in which patient bodies are physically controlled and managed. Panoptic power has been associated with the ability of the individual to freely participate in changing their behaviour through subtle processes (Foucault, 1979). There is therefore a gap between nursing care practices based on sovereign power and the disciplinary aspect of panoptic power. When the patient is inside the ward, it is not only sufficient to control their behaviour, but they also have to accept that they have a mental health condition (see Chapter 2). The ward, therefore, is not only reliant on sovereign power and panoptic power in shaping patient behaviour, but pastoral power also plays a significant part in how the patient is disciplined inside the ward. Pastoral power in the context of the power held by the patient's consultant psychiatrist has received less attention in the governance of patients inside the ward. Its significance lies in how patients can negotiate their recovery, or come to an agreement about their recovery, with their consultant psychiatrist in exchange for their discharge from the ward. However, before moving on to explore this in more detail, it is useful to examine how the cameras as a means of panoptic surveillance shape the patient experience inside the mental health ward.

Foucault's (1979: 201) panopticism was reliant on the visibility of those being watched and the invisibility of those doing the watching, where according to Foucault Bentham's Panopticon:

> laid down the principle that power should be visible and unverifiable. Visible: the inmate will constantly have before his [*sic*] eyes the tall outline of the central tower from which he [*sic*] is spied. Unverifiable: the inmate must never know whether he is being looked at any one moment.

However, inside all three PICUs, not only were patients visible, so were the staff who were watching them. Foucault (1979: 201–202) describes Bentham's central tower as having:

> venetian blinds on the windows of the central observation hall, but, on the inside, partitions that intersected the hall at right angles and, in order to pass from one quarter to another, not doors but zig-zag openings; for the slightest noise, a gleam of light, a brightness in a half-opened door would betray the presence of the guardian ... in the peripheric ring, one is totally seen, without ever seeing; in the central tower, one sees everything without ever being seen.

Architecturally, it was the ward office that physically and metaphorically represented the central tower described by Foucault. The ward office held a central location where staff could view patients in most parts of the communal areas of the ward, along the male and female corridors and various other spaces, such as dining areas, activity rooms and patient lounge areas. However, unlike Foucault's central tower, all three PICUs shared similar design features in relation to their openness. Glass windows surrounded the ward office, and glass panels inside ward office doors exposed staff inside them. Patients could look into the ward office and know who was in there and staff could look out of the office, easily surveilling large parts of the ward and patients inside them. This representation of the central tower is very different from Foucault's (1979) description. Even though patients and staff were not informed about camera use inside the ward, the use of cameras was not hidden from them. For example, several patients and most agency and bank staff knew that the ward used CCTV because as well as the cameras inside the ward, they could see CCTV monitors inside the ward office.

CCTV monitors were not only visible inside the ward office. Monitors inside the seclusion area and bedroom cameras were also exposed. In their use in seclusion, for example, CCTV monitors were not discreetly hidden inside the seclusion lobby. The monitors were attached to a wall directly opposite the window panel which separated the seclusion room from the seclusion lobby. This meant that patients could see the CCTV monitor and their image on it. Although they were not told about the camera in seclusion, they could see the monitor and knew that the ward used CCTV to monitor them. Some patients in seclusion were also aware that even when staff closed the blind restricting their direct vision into the seclusion room, they were still being monitored by them via the CCTV monitor in the seclusion lobby. Therefore, while patients and staff were not explicitly informed about the cameras, several patients and most staff were aware that the ward used cameras. Patients also knew that staff used the cameras to watch them. Also, most patients were not surprised that the ward had cameras. The practice inside all three PICUs to give patients an admission information sheet explicitly telling them that they were in the ward to be observed meant that most patients assumed that the cameras were there to watch them and not staff.

Watching of patients was not limited to CCTV camera use. The primary form of monitoring patients in the ward was by either hourly (inside two PICUs) or half-hourly (inside one PICU) nurse observation of patients. Although some staff did use the cameras to sign off patients as having been observed, most monitoring of patients tended to be face-to-face observations. Nurse observations were staggered so that patients did not always know when their next nurse observation would happen. Holmes (2001) describes how the panoptic nature of nurse observations is reliant on the patient not knowing when the nurse will next come to view them. According to him, it is this uncertainty as to when they might be looked at again which results in the panoptic gaze and the shaping of patient behaviour. CCTV cameras have also been associated with the panoptic gaze and in the self-regulation of behaviour where the central tower is replaced by the cameras creating uncertainty of watching. However, the cameras inside the ward were not used in the same way. Most patients knew the cameras were inside the ward to watch them, and they were aware that staff used them to observe them. This is because they could look into the ward office and watch staff and know if they were looking at the CCTV monitor. Most patients knew that the cameras were not watched continuously because they could see that there was no staff sat next to the CCTV monitor looking at it. Although the cameras did create a level of uncertainty as to when the staff might use them for observation, most patients were not too worried by this. In addition, by using the cameras to do nurse observations (see Chapter 4), staff undermined the panoptic aspect of face-to-face nurse observations as described by Holmes (2001).

The visibility of the real cameras did however lead several patients to believe that the ward also had hidden cameras. Even those patients who were well enough to leave the PICU (and therefore having the mental capacity to understand the purpose of the cameras) imagined that there were likely to be hidden cameras inside it. These patients also believed that camera footage and live feeds were regularly viewed by their consultant psychiatrist, including footage and live feeds linked to hidden cameras. It was in the context of hidden cameras that Foucault's (1979) metaphor of the Panopticon was probably most relevant in affecting patient behaviour. Several patients pointed out smoke alarms, sprinklers and various other gadgets inside their bedroom and in communal areas of the ward as examples of hidden cameras, including inside those bedrooms which had real cameras in them. Patients deployed a range of tactics, including some which also undermined ward safety. For example, by pulling apart, hitting or attempting to smear food, or other liquids, such as shaving foam, liquid soap and hand cream. In this way, patients damaged fire alarms and other safety features. Inside all three PICUs, the transparency of the ward office and the visibility of staff operated as a reminder to patients that they were always under surveillance. This led patients to believe that they were under observation even when they were not, leading them to conform their behaviour as if they were being watched through, what Norris and Armstrong (1999) describe as "anticipatory conformity".

Unlike the real cameras which could easily be seen inside the ward, most patients did not feel as though they were in control of hidden cameras. For example, P12 (Chapter 5) effectively describes how even the simple act of pacing in his bedroom becomes a problematic activity as he does not know how this behaviour will be judged by others. Other patients preferred not to sleep in their bedroom and be in full view of real cameras, and one patient often slept under his bed to avoid hidden cameras (Field note: 118). Also, several patients could not describe or explain how staff and their consultant psychiatrist would judge what would be normal behaviour for them. For these patients, it was not the real cameras that were necessarily the source of their stress. The real cameras functioned to stabilise the activity of constant observation of patients inside the ward. This activity was not based on leaving patients as subjects of surveillance, guessing whether they were being watched or not. It was about exposing the gaze so that patients were under no doubt that they were always looked at. According to Foucault (1979), discipline is a mechanism of power that regulates the thoughts and behaviours of people through subtle processes. However, the belief that all their behaviour was under constant scrutiny left several patients feeling uneasy. They struggled to conform their behaviour to what was expected of them because they were unsure what normal behaviour inside the ward should look like. Most patients worried that anything they did would be judged negatively by staff.

Sovereign power, panoptic power, pastoral power

According to Foucault (1979), the operation of power requires the exposure of bodies in three significant ways. This includes bodies as targets of surveillance, expert knowledge and corrective measures. Central to disciplinary power Foucault believed was the examination. The examination is the combination of panoptic observation and normalising judgement. Patients inside the mental health hospital have to be classified (with a mental disorder or having a mental disorder that has yet to be categorised), sorted and differentiated (often through age, gender, type of disorder and the risk that they pose). Inside the ward, the examination of the patient body as a target for surveillance has importance because it shows whether the patient has "reached the level required" for recovery, through the process of being involved in treatment. For this to happen, the examination of each patient's body also requires "differentiating the abilities of each individual" (Foucault, 1979: 158). This form of power Foucault suggests is a form of power that cannot be exercised without knowing the inside of people's minds and "without exploring their souls". It also "implies a knowledge of the conscience and an ability to direct it". This hierarchical power is invested in the body of the consultant psychiatrist (through pastoral power). It is, according to Foucault,

> salvation oriented (as opposed to political power). It is oblative (as opposed to the principle of sovereignty); it is individualizing (as opposed to legal power); it is coextensive and continuous with life; it is linked with a production of truth.
>
> (Foucault cited in Dreyfus and Rabinow, 1983: 214)

Pastoral power therefore is not concerned with day-to-day management of the ward and the conflict between patients and staff or staff and managers. It is solely concerned with the well-being of the patient and the ability to cure or conform the patient's conduct so that they no longer need the mental health hospital any more.

Although the consultant psychiatrist spent very little time inside the ward, their absence did not mean that they were forgotten. When patients did meet with their consultant psychiatrist, this was often during weekly multidisciplinary meetings, where the patient would not necessarily be alone with the consultant but would be seen alongside a range of other clinical practitioners who may or may not be responsible for the patient's care. In all three PICUs, the consultant psychiatrist was not involved in the day-to-day problems linked to patient care; they were more interested in factors such as the circumstances that led to the patient being inside the ward. These included aiming to understand why a patient is disruptive, why they might not be sleeping well and any other circumstances surrounding a patient's mental health condition. This was so that they could better understand the patient's disorder and help them towards their recovery. Information about the patient was provided by nursing staff, junior doctors or registrars and the patient's family. The consultant psychiatrist had very little contact with the patient who may or may not have differing views from those offered by nurses, their family and other healthcare workers. It was therefore the consultant psychiatrist's positioning in the ward, through authority invested in the visibility of their body and their ability to control the patient's destiny, which resulted in panoptic disciplinary surveillance. This is very similar to Moore's (2011) analysis of courtroom judges, where the site of power is visible in the body of the judge as an authority. Therefore, patients were only partially interested in seeking approval from ward staff, as they were more interested in gaining approval from their consultant psychiatrist.

It was the panoptic aspect of the consultant psychiatrist's individualising power that maintained hierarchy inside the ward. Inside research sites 1 and 2, each PICU had a dedicated consultant psychiatrist. These consultant psychiatrists would not have known the patients very well as most patients would have been transferred from another ward. This meant that they would have been under the care of a different consultant, or they would have been detained inside the ward from the community. Therefore, most patients would also not have known the consultant psychiatrist inside the PICU. The lack of private contact with their consultant psychiatrist meant that some patients believed that staff, especially nursing staff, did not always provide their consultant with accurate information about their conduct inside the ward. For these patients, the cameras became a significant point of contact with their consultant psychiatrist. They believed that CCTV footage showing their ability to control their behaviour in the ward was being analysed by their consultant or was likely to be seen by their consultant, although they were not always sure. Most patients believed that the cameras must be seen by someone; otherwise, there was no reason to have them. They, therefore, surmised that camera footage was seen by their consultant, as one patient commented similar to their consultant looking at them through a two-way mirror. For these patients, the supervisor/guardian in the panoptic tower was not the staff but their consultant psychiatrist. Even though they remained unsure whether their consultant viewed CCTV footage or not, they aimed to conduct their behaviour as if they did. This was so that they could directly prove to them that they were ready for discharge. These patients not only understood the hierarchical nature of the consultant psychiatrist's power and their ability to discharge them from the ward, they also saw the cameras as a direct link to their consultant, by-passing ward staff whom some patients did not always trust. It was in their ability to maintain their individualising power in this way that the cameras were most effective in shaping patient conduct.

This panoptic aspect of the individualising power of the consultant psychiatrist was also present inside research site 3. This PICU did not have a consultant psychiatrist at the ward lead. This ward had a nurse consultant lead. Each patient maintained a link with their consultant psychiatrist, rather than their case being passed onto a PICU consultant psychiatrist. The reasoning behind this was so that patients can have a continuation in their care from the same consultant psychiatrist. However, inside sites 1 and 2, there were times when the consultant psychiatrist entered the ward for other reasons than the weekly multidisciplinary meeting. For example, inside site 2, the consultant psychiatrist spent half a day inside the ward office doing administrative work and catching up with staff, where he was visible to patients. He also attended and sometimes chaired patient and staff weekly meetings. There was no such presence of the consultant psychiatrist inside site 3, and this made patients nervous, especially as they were unsure about what information was shared about them to their consultant by the staff. Although several patients inside all three PICUs believed that their consultant psychiatrist looked at live feeds and recorded footage of their conduct inside the ward, inside site 3, this belief in the real and imagined hidden cameras was felt more intensely. It was in the panoptic aspect of the individualising power of the consultant psychiatrist, their ability to control the destiny of each patient and their interest in each patient, which resulted in the PICU becoming a panoptic machine. It did not matter whether the patient believed that they were royalty or God as part of their delusional belief. What mattered was their ability to not share these thoughts openly and aim to conduct their behaviour in ways that showed others, but especially their consultant psychiatrist that they could control their urge not to behave like royalty. In this way, the PICU also became a curing machine because the cameras, both real and imagined hidden ones, also became a conduit by which patients became docile bodies. This aspect of the panoptic individualising power of the consultant psychiatrist and other authority figures has received little attention in surveillance literature, especially in the shaping of people's conduct.

In carrying out the task of clinical observations, some staff also used the cameras to watch patients in those parts of the ward that had cameras in them so that they could learn more about each patient. This use of cameras was based on bettering their understanding of each patient and the stimulation and risk triggers of these patients so that they could engage with them more productively. This use of CCTV was not motivated by the desire to belittle, mock or expose the behaviour of the patient; it was a genuine attempt to understand their behaviour so that they could respond positively to it. This need to understand how their behaviour changes when they are unwell was also something that interested some patients. For example, during fieldwork observations, there was a patient who told me that he would like to see CCTV footage of himself when he is unwell to gain a better understanding of how his behaviour changed (Field note: 225). He claimed that although his wife and others around him described how his behaviour changes, he wanted to see this for himself to understand why he continuously ends up in the hospital under detention. Rose (1989: 11) claims that it is through "self-inspection, self-problematization, self-monitoring and confession" that we learn to "evaluate ourselves according to the criteria provided for us by others", and in this regard, the use of cameras in enabling patients in the process of "normalising" their behaviour was perceived by few patients and some staff as a useful tool. In societies of control, Deleuze (1992: 5) argues individuals are no longer going from one closed site to another such as from the mental health hospital to the family, because "one is never finished with anything". This development suggests that the consultant psychiatrist is no longer required to enlist the support of other people in the disciplining of the patient's behaviour as the patient becomes more proficient at governing themselves not only through self-monitoring practices but also by becoming efficient at developing their expertise and understanding about medical interventions. This promotes the rise of synoptic surveillance practices through the process of self-examination, which, for some patients, begins inside the ward.

Foucault (cited in Gordon, 1980) believed that repressive power is limited by its prohibitive force, and, therefore, for power to be effective, it has to be productive. CCTV cameras were also used in the production of knowledge about each patient. For instance, in all three wards, it was common practice to review incidents in the ward where repressive force was used (for example, in a full-body restraint) so that staff could learn how to handle future altercations with patients better. Where this was available, CCTV footage was used to enable this learning. Some staff also used the cameras to better understand a patient for whom they were a key worker. In all three PICUs, each patient was allocated a keyworker (staff member), who changed each shift. Patients could approach their keyworker if they needed additional emotional support. The role of the keyworker staff is to produce a report of the patient, for whom they are an allocated keyworker, at the end of their shift. While this practice is essentially about documented surveillance practice, it was based on the principle of individualised care of each patient which recognises that all patients have different emotional needs. In this respect, keyworkers were keen to understand the emotions and behaviour of their particular patient during each shift and at staff handover meetings. These practices were designed around ensuring the individuality of each patient, where Foucault (2009) claims that pastoral care also extends to each sheep. Sovereign power, panoptic power and pastoral power were, therefore, used in varying degrees by staff and the patient's consultant psychiatrist to discipline patient behaviour inside the ward. Staff had access to a range of techniques, including those based on sovereign power (such as the use of seclusion, forced medication), panoptic power (through nurse observation practices) and pastoral power (as a keyworker) in their ability to assist the consultant psychiatrist and enable patient recovery. Similarly, the consultant psychiatrist held ultimate sovereign power in their ability to discharge the patient from the ward. They continue to hold this unique position despite the amendment of the 1983 Mental Health Act in 2007 (in England and Wales) enabling any other health professional to assume clinical responsibility to discharge patients from the mental health ward. This is because no other mental health professional would undermine the decision of the consultant psychiatrist if the consultant believed that a patient was not ready for discharge from the ward. It was their ability to decide the patient's destiny (whether they could be discharged from the ward) and their authority embodied in their individualising power which was the most productive in shaping the patient's conduct.

Implications for practice

Background

In the post-institutional era, the availability of surveillance technologies (such as CCTV) not only allows the modern mental health hospital to stand apart from asylums but also offers new ways of monitoring patients inside the ward. The empirical data for this research has already identified how CCTV influences staff and patient relationships inside the ward. For example, through the reduction and sometimes the loss of face-to-face contact with patients, the overexposure of patient bodies and in the medical analysing of patient behaviours by being able to observe the patient unobtrusively. Research data has also shown that CCTV cameras are not tools that are used by staff (and sometimes managers) when the occasional need arises. Staff used the cameras to change the way that they carry out the task of nursing or healthcare work inside the ward (see Chapter 4). As a result, the cameras did influence practices inside the ward because they provided a solution to criticism about the care of patients. This criticism is not only evident from outside sources, for example, in the televising of documentaries by BBC 1 Panorama programmes (2019, 2011) (see Chapter 2 for more detail). Nursing and mental health literature are also critical about patient care and staff safety inside wards (Kanvera, 2012; Bowers, 2014; d'Ettore and Pelliciani, 2017). Managers, therefore, attempted to seek local solutions to what are essentially national political concerns related to poor resourcing, management and organisation of mental health services. For some managers, even though there had been no local concern, the potential for any future problems that may bring about negative publicity to their organisation was reason enough to install cameras inside the ward. The second part of this chapter highlights three practice concerns and their implications for patients in the use of CCTV cameras inside the ward.

Criminalisation of patients

The presence of cameras inside the ward was not a surprise to most staff; they expected an intensive care unit to have cameras inside it because they assumed that most patients inside these wards would be violent and difficult to manage. Kasmi (2007: 75), for example, describes a typical PICU patient as a:

> young schizophrenic detained male, belonging to an ethnic minority (if in an inner city), known to mental health services with previous informal, detained and PICU admissions, admitted due to violence and often possessing a forensic history. If a complex need existed, it was usually substance misuse. The inpatient stay tended to be for less than two months and discharge was usually to an acute ward.

Haggerty and Ericson (2007) suggest that the expansion of surveillance is dependent on its ability to cohere with other agendas. There were several reasons why managers believed that the cameras were useful to the ward environment. For example, the idea that the cameras could create a better risk-free ward environment was one of the appeals of the cameras for managers who were unsure how to respond to violent situations inside them. Most managers did not believe that the cameras would deter patient violence. This is because, according to them, those patients who did become violent often did so when they did not have the full mental capacity to control their behaviour and, therefore, did not necessarily understand what they were doing. These managers did not believe that the Department of Health policies, such as "zero tolerance" to violence, could be successfully implemented inside mental health wards (DH, 1999). However, despite this, site 2 decided to increase the number of cameras in the ward following an incident in which a member of staff was injured while carrying out their job and blamed the organisation for their injury. The expansion of surveillance was therefore not always limited to the creation of a better ward environment for patients and staff. For some managers, the expansion of surveillance was linked to protecting the reputation of the organisation and the need to reduce litigation disputes. These disputes resulted not only in the loss of money through compensation but also in the loss of labour, as the staff who are injured require time off work to recover.

Several managers believed that the camera's potential for providing additional evidence in resolving disputes and in reducing compensation claims made them invaluable. This was their belief even when the cameras were not successful in resolving disputes because the incident was not captured on camera, or what was captured was of insufficient quality, or did not show the whole incident. The justification for their continued use and the addition of more cameras was based on their potential to resolve these matters. It was therefore the camera's potential to bring about order inside the ward that had appeal for managers. Some managers, therefore, believed that the cameras enabled them to be orientated inside the ward, even when they could not physically be there. Also, the cameras enabled them to discriminate between different accounts of what happened when an incident did take place. These managers did not view the use of cameras in this way to enforce their hierarchical position inside the ward. They were keen to learn from incidents to create a more stable ward environment. This done well has the potential to integrate the group, including those individuals who have perhaps not acted according to what is expected of them.

The availability of CCTV recordings to provide evidence when a violent incident has happened inside the ward resulted in the expectation by some staff that this would lead to serious consequences for those patients carrying out violent acts. Inside one PICU, the assaultive behaviour of a patient led to staff and managers reporting the patient to the police on three separate occasions. This patient (see Chapter 4) had been removed from the ward and detained inside a police station as a result of his assaultive behaviour towards staff and another patient. On one occasion, part of the assault was captured on camera. Staff believed that this evidence, together with their verbal accounts, should have resulted in a police prosecution of the patient. This is because, in addition to their verbal accounts, there was also visual evidence of the part capture of the patient assaulting staff. These staff believed that the correct action for the police should be to prosecute the patient because the cameras had provided evidence, and the patient should be held accountable for their behaviour. In this way, the cameras were not just a black box providing managers and staff with information about what was happening inside the ward; they also became a means by which already existing pressures inside the ward were exposed. In this example, the reporting to the police of the patient's assaultive behaviour has serious consequences for the patient in ways that he might not have imagined when he was detained inside the ward. That is, if the police had prosecuted him, he would be leaving the mental health ward with a criminal record. Or his care would be escalated to a secure care ward where he would have to spend a longer period in hospital. This use of the cameras also has the potential to marginalise those people who are already discriminated against because of their mental health status. The further criminalisation of the patient at a time when they are seriously ill and deemed unable to live in society, the ability of the cameras to provide additional evidence for criminal prosecution has serious implications for any patient entering the mental health hospital. It also raises serious concerns about mental health nursing practices, therapeutic interventions and questions the primary function of the mental health hospital.

Gender and surveillance

The issue regarding gender and camera use also created a range of safeguarding concerns related to women's mental health care. The abuse of women inside mental health wards is not only limited to sexual and physical abuse. Nicki (2001) also describes how the use of language and the problematisation of women's behaviour can lead to discriminatory responses to women. Inside two PICUs, some women patients kept removing their clothing. This behaviour was related to their mental health condition. One of these women also engaged in sexualised behaviour with other patients and was sometimes also sexually inappropriate with male staff. This patient was placed in seclusion as her sexual advances towards other patients were perceived as a threat to male patients who, because of their mental health status, were also deemed to be vulnerable. Although seclusion is not the ideal solution, it did, to some extent, protect the female patient because it physically removed her from those patients and staff who could also take advantage of her. It also stopped her from getting agitated and aggressive with staff when they attempted to stop her from removing her clothes. While some staff believed that this was appropriate action to protect her, they did not always understand how the continuous view of her, often seen naked on the CCTV monitor inside the ward office, was inappropriate. Not only this, but it also led to staff being critical about her behaviour and recalling incidents about how she attempted to be promiscuous with male staff or vulnerable male patients (see Chapter 4). It was the exposure of her naked body to staff in the ward office via the CCTV monitor which was a safeguarding issue. This is because it changed the nature of her relationship with staff, how she was judged by them and how she was seen. In this way, the camera inside the seclusion room did not submissively pass information from one space to another, that is, the seclusion room to the ward office. It was also responsible for a set of values, which Ellul (1964) suggests left ignored or unrecognised impose themselves on staff and the relationships that they form with patients.

Similarly, inside research site 3, the female-only ward area was covered by cameras and the male-only ward area was not covered by any cameras. Women patients could be watched while they were sleeping through infrared cameras; they could be seen on CCTV monitors as they left their bedroom area and entered the women-only lounge area. The only place that they could not be seen by cameras was in the communal area where they spent most time of their time. Some managers believed that increased surveillance of women patients through the addition of more cameras in women-only ward areas was necessary to protect them. According to Bordo (1993), women therefore not only have to be disciplined in relation to their madness, but their bodies also have to be regulated according to societal expectations that are dominated by male expectations. In September 2002, the Department of Health launched the document *Women's Mental Health: Into the Mainstream*. The recommendation that women should have their own separate mental healthcare service was a key conclusion of this document. However, the financial implications of having separate services for women patients has meant that most mental health hospitals have interpreted separation of women's mental health care into separate male and female areas inside the ward. This Department of Health document and others have also emphasised how women's mental health should be addressed differently (see, for example, Abel and Newbigging, 2018; Department of Health and Social Care, 2018). However, the data for this research suggests that apart from the separation of sleeping accommodation, responses by staff and managers to certain behaviours by women were largely unsatisfactory. For example, inside site 1, staff believed that it was appropriate to manage a woman's promiscuous behaviour by placing her in seclusion, while inside site 3, managers believed that women's vulnerability inside the ward should be managed by more CCTV surveillance and exposure of their bodies.

The exposure of women's bodies, especially when they are displaying disinhibited behaviour, was also not perceived by staff as a safeguarding issue under the Care Act (2014). This left women patients who did engage in disinhibited behaviours vulnerable in two ways. First, whether women patients knowingly engaged in sexualised behaviour or whether their sexualised behaviour was associated with their mental health condition, this behaviour left them open to abuse inside the ward. For example, similar to daytime observations when staff were doing night-time observations using bedroom cameras, they are working alone. Therefore, they are looking at some women patients engaging in a wide range of sexualised behaviour with no other staff or managers policing what they are watching. At night-time, the number of staff available on shift is significantly reduced, which means that the ward was often empty. When a staff member operates the bedroom CCTV monitor, there is no record of how long they spent looking at the patient in their bedroom, and because bedroom cameras are live feeds only, there is no recording of what they were observing. As the monitoring is undertaken by a lone staff member, there is no other staff around to question why they spent longer looking at a particular patient. This makes the patient vulnerable because it leaves them open to the voyeuristic gaze. Some people may argue that it is not necessarily the bedroom cameras that make women vulnerable in this way and also that women are also left vulnerable through in-person observation. However, as already discussed (see Chapter 3), in a face-to-face encounter, the staff member doing the watching is also looked at by the patient and therefore has to confront their feelings about their behaviour and know that they have also been seen (Lyon, 1994).

Secondly, Soomar and Ali (2017) identify a range of disinhibited sexualised behaviours, which, they claim, patients with certain mental disorders, including dementia, schizophrenia and anxiety disorders, are apt to engage in. They propose a behavioural model of intervention which is about diverting this behaviour. However, in the two PICUs that had women patients inside them who engaged in disinhibited sexualised behaviour, staff responses did not appear to reflect this. In research site 1, the woman patient was placed in seclusion, and in site 2, the woman patient was allowed to wander around the ward often without supervision. During fieldwork observations, the female patient in site 2 was seen topless in front of male patients on two occasions and completely naked in front of a workman with no staff monitoring her behaviour. Both these behaviours were in the communal areas of the ward where there should have been staff present and where there were CCTV cameras. In these situations, the cameras did not protect vulnerable women patients; they instead opened up other ways to extend the voyeuristic gaze by exposing women's bodies inside the seclusion room, inside their bedroom and in communal areas of the ward.

Ethical practice

In their review of CCTV camera use inside mental health wards, Appenzeller and Appelbaum (2020: 480) suggest that the main ethical conflict related to camera use is in the balancing of "patient's autonomy and privacy" against "patient and staff security and safety". This research suggests that although having privacy inside the ward was a concern for many patients, for example, Chapter 5 explores how patients attempted to neutralise surveillance inside the ward to gain privacy, privacy alone was less concerning than how the cameras impacted on ethical mental healthcare practices inside the ward. For example, the cameras were not placed inside the ward so that they could be used to make negative judgements about patients. However, their presence inside the ward and their ability to see patients in ways that they might not otherwise be seen allowed staff to make judgements that were not always positive (see Chapter 4). During fieldwork observations when staff looked at CCTV monitors inside the ward office or seclusion room, it was often to make negative statements about patient behaviour. This was opposite to how they spoke about or interacted with patients when they were engaged in face-to-face conversation with them.

Several staff, for example, when talking to or talking about patients in communal areas of the ward, often said positive things about them. These face-to-face encounters in the communal areas of the ward sometimes led to a genuine conversation between the staff and patient. For example, a female staff member reminded a female patient about how she had deeply scratched, bitten and spat at her when she was first admitted to the ward. She would show the patient a scratch on her arm which was still healing. The patient responded by apologising to her and letting her know that she was embarrassed by her behaviour and that she was sorry. This exposure of the patient's behaviour when she was acutely unwell was not done to belittle or upset her; it was done to genuinely help the patient recognise how she behaves when she is unwell. While this was a difficult encounter, the ability of the staff to confront the patient face-to-face allowed the patient to respond to her. This encounter was ethical because of the honesty and openness of the conversation. This is far more effective than showing someone recorded images of how they look when they are not well. Even though the confrontation of the encounter between the staff and patient was uncomfortable, it was the genuineness of the interaction which was therapeutic for both the patient and the staff, who had been at the receiving end of the patient's violent behaviour. This suggests that working with people with mental health conditions is a skilled task which requires skilled workers who have the ability to interact with patients openly and honestly.

Inside all three PICUs involved in the research, there was no clear purpose for camera use inside communal areas of the ward. According to most managers, the cameras were not prioritised inside the ward because they were a useful management tool and neither were they placed inside the ward to enable staff to do nursing more efficiently. The only exception was bedroom cameras, where there was a clear purpose for their use and patients had a right to refuse to be monitored by them during the night. Several managers believed that the cameras protected the rights of staff and patients inside the ward, although how they did this was not explained to them. Therefore, the presence of cameras made both patients and staff believe that their actions and behaviour inside the ward was perceived by others as being untrustworthy. For example, during fieldwork observations, several patients linked camera use to wrongdoing. This wrongdoing was often linked to their behaviour and not the behaviour of the staff. Therefore, patients did not believe that the cameras would exonerate them in a volatile situation. The lack of clarity in the introduction of the cameras to the ward environment and in their uses inside the ward also meant that there was no limitation around how the cameras could be used. On one hand, some managers believed that it was appropriate to expand the use of cameras. For example, to monitor authorised leave for patients outside the hospital periphery expanding the use of cameras immediately outside the PICU (Chapter 5), or by adding more cameras to the ward environment after an incident. However, when staff wanted to expand camera use in opening up of hot-spot areas of the ward (see Chapters 4 and 5), this use of cameras was resisted by managers. It was therefore unclear what managers intended in their use of cameras and how any use was justified and explained to staff. This was the case even though each NHS Trust made a local decision to introduce cameras into the ward environment.

Most managers and staff regarded the cameras as a security feature even though staff used the cameras to carry out certain nursing tasks inside the ward. It was not always easy to identify who had responsibility for the cameras inside the ward. Staff and managers ultimately named the Chief Executive of the NHS Trust as having the final responsibility. However, on a day-to-day basis, most staff and managers remained unsure. This affected how staff carried out nursing practices inside the ward in two significant ways. First, there was no internal evaluation as to how the cameras were being used by staff. Although the PICUs and NHS Trust had procedures to assess the use of CCTV cameras within hospital grounds, there were no equivalent processes or procedures for evaluating camera use inside the ward. Second, the lack of clarity around who was responsible for the cameras meant that there was no one monitoring how the cameras were used as part of day-to-day nursing care inside the ward. Several staff believed that the cameras were a useful tool in how they did their job. However, as this research has shown, the ability to distance themselves from other colleagues and managers using CCTV monitors did not always lead to positive talk about them. This was not surprising as the cameras promoted an ethical stance inside the ward which was about establishing guilt and promoting suspicion. In this way, CCTV technology stood in direct opposition to the ethical principle of mental health care based on establishing relationships with patients and showing compassion. It was therefore not surprising that staff looked at CCTV monitors in order to highlight and identify patient behaviours, peer behaviours and manager behaviours that were problematic. However, in doing so, the cameras undermined ethical mental health practice.

The negative ethical stance promoted by cameras also influenced how patients behaved inside the ward and how they perceived staff. Patients also felt that the cameras were inside the ward to negatively judge them. As a result, some patients found the cameras very intrusive. In this way, the cameras did not open up spaces inside the ward. They had an opposite effect. For example, the belief that they were under constant observation meant that patients struggled to find spaces inside the ward where they believed there were no cameras and where they could be themselves without feeling under continuous observation. Most patients were unsure where the cameras were located inside each PICU. There was no signage, for example, inside any of the three PICUs, alerting patients to the fact that a particular area was covered by CCTV cameras. This left some patients believing that all areas were covered by cameras, and it also raised suspicion about hidden cameras. Inside one PICU, there was no camera inside the lounge room. However, there was a camera located directly outside the room which captured images of the garden/courtyard area that could be easily seen from the window in the lounge room. The location of the camera in this way meant that several patients believed that it also captured images inside the lounge room even though it did not. This stopped some patients from using this area as they believed that they would be monitored by the cameras. These experiences impacted on how patients behaved inside the ward, and it also influenced how staff interpreted their behaviour. These examples suggest that camera use inside mental health wards also need to consider how they influence ethical mental health practice. In order to do this effectively, any review of camera use inside the ward needs to start from an ethical standpoint which promotes ethical mental health practice.

Final word

On theory

Surveillance literature has tended to emphasise Foucault's (1979) analysis of Bentham's Panopticon in the analysis of CCTV cameras. It is the uncertainty of not knowing when one is being looked at which creates compliance of behaviour. In this research, I have shown that the mental health ward is different. Not only are the cameras and CCTV monitors visible to patients, but the patient also knows that staff use them to watch them. This is because they know that they are inside the ward to be observed. It was the knowledge that they were under observation inside the ward and the absence of their consultant psychiatrist which led several patients inside all three PICUs to believe that their consultant psychiatrist might be watching live or recorded footage through real and imagined hidden cameras. It was this uncertainty of their consultant psychiatrist who may or may not be watching them which led to anticipatory conformity of patients inside the ward.

To date, there has been little analysis of the individualising power invested in the authority of certain figures such as the consultant psychiatrist in the analysis of panoptic surveillance. Although Foucault examines the individualising power of the consultant psychiatrist in the context of pastoral power, he does not link this to panoptic power and sovereign power. In my practice as a social worker, although I perceived my job as mostly about keeping families together, it was the legal authority that I held, that is, the ability to remove a child from her family, which was also central to compliance from a person or the family that I worked with. The panoptic nature of this individualising power was in the not knowing what information I had about the family and, if and when the child might be removed.

This research has highlighted the need to examine the panoptic authority invested in bodies of people who hold legal positional power such as the consultant psychiatrist, social worker, police and courtroom judges. It is their ability to change an individual's circumstances through legal power that creates docile bodies. In addition, clients, service users and people also resist surveillance from social workers, police and courtroom judges, and currently, very little is known about how they do this. Therefore, influencing the conduct of people is not limited to the hospital, prison or the courtroom. It extends beyond these structures through the authority invested in the bodies of certain individuals who hold legal power. It is this aspect of caring surveillance which remains underexplored. This surveillance is also not always experienced negatively by people who are at the receiving end of it. This is because although there are legal implications linked to conformity, it is how well the social worker, police, consultant psychiatrist or courtroom judge uses their power to bring about conformity, that is, without resorting to removing any child from their family, or detaining a person inside a mental health hospital, or sending a person to prison, as to how they measure their success.

On practice

As a final word, there are three linked points to CCTV camera use inside mental health wards which I would like to reiterate. First, empirical data for this research has drawn attention to how the perception of increased violence inside mental health wards has the potential to criminalise the patient. This is done to patients at a time when they are not always in a position to control their emotions. Therefore, mental health hospitals have to decide whether it is the criminalisation of the patient which is their priority or patient recovery and change the ward environment to reflect this. Second, the exposure of women's naked bodies and their sexualised behaviours, whether this was in their bedroom, in seclusion or corridor and communal spaces, requires a serious response. While some staff and managers were concerned about this, there was a general acceptance that this behaviour is part of their mental health condition about which little can be done. This behaviour places women patients in a vulnerable situation inside the ward and is a safeguarding concern where the cameras do not protect women, but instead increase their surveillance and constitutes yet another means by which they can be potentially abused. Finally, the lack of an overarching ethical approach to camera implementation, rationale and their uses inside the ward has meant that the cameras have and can be used to undermine the underlying principles and values of professional mental healthcare practice.

Bibliography

Abel, K. and Newbigging, K. (2018). *Addressing Unmet Needs in Women's Mental Health*, Tavistock Square, London: British Medical Association.

Appenzeller, Y.E. and Appelbaum, P.S. (2020). "Ethical and practical issues in video surveillance of psychiatric units," *Psychiatric Services*, 71(5): 480–486.

Bijker, W.E., Hughes, T.P. and Pinch, T. (eds) (2012). *The Social Construction of Technological Systems*, 2nd edition, Cambridge MA: MIT Press.

Bordo, S. (1993). *Unbearable Weight: Feminism, Western Culture and the Body*, Berkeley: University of California.

Bowers, L. (2014). "Safewards: A new model of conflict and containment on psychiatric wards," *Journal of Psychiatric and Mental Health Nursing*, 21(6): 499–508.

British Broadcasting Company (BBC 1). *Undercover Care: The Abuse Exposed, Winterbourne View*, Panorama, 31 May 2011.

British Broadcasting Company (BBC 1). *Undercover Hospital Abuse Scandal, Whorlton Hall*, Panorama, 22 May 2019.

Cuchetti, C. and Grace, P.J. (2020). "Authentic intention: Tempering the dehumanizing aspects of technology on behalf of good nursing care," *Nursing Philosophy*, 21(1). Available online: https://onlinelibrary.wiley.com [accessed 21 June 2021].

Department of Health (DH). (1999). *Campaign to Stop Violence against Staff Working in the NHS: NHS Zero Tolerance HSC 1999/226*, London: Department of Health.

Department of Health (DH). (2002). *Women's Mental Health: Into the Mainstream Strategic Development for Mental Health Care for Women*, London: Department of Health.

Department of Health and Social Care. (2018). *Time to Change*. Mind and Rethink Mental Illness. Available online: www.time-to-change.org.uk [accessed 10 October 2018].

Deleuze, G. (1992). "Postscript on the societies of control," *October*, 59: 3–7

d' Ettorre, G. and Pellicani, V. (2017). "Workplace violence toward mental healthcare workers employed in psychiatric wards," *Safety and Health at Work*, 8(4): 337–342.

Dreyfus, H.L. and Rabinow, P. (1983). *Michel Foucault: Beyond Structuralism and Hermeneutics. 2nd edition. With an Afterword by an Interview with Michel Foucault*, Chicago: The University of Chicago Press.

Ellul, J. (1964). *The Technological Society*, New York: Vintage Books.

Foucault, M. (1979). *Discipline and Punish: The Birth of the Prison*, New York: Vintage.

Foucault, M. (2008). *Psychiatric Power: Lectures at the Collège de France 1973–1974*, edited by Jacques Lagrange and translated by Graham Burchell, Basingstoke: Palgrave.

Foucault, M. (2009). *Security, Territory, Population: Lectures at the Collège de France 1977–1978*, edited by Michel Senellart and translated by Graham Burchell, Basinstoke: Palgrave.

Gordon, C. (ed) (1980). *Michel Foucault: Power/Knowledge. Selected Interviews and Other Writings 1972–1977 By Michel Foucault*, translated by C. Gordon, L. Marshall, J. Mepham and K. Soper, New York: Harvester Wheatsheaf.

Haggerty, K.D. and Ericson, R.V. (eds) (2007). *The New Politics Surveillance and Visibility*, Toronto, Buffalo, London: University of Toronto Press.

Hand, S. (1997). *Difficult Freedom: Essay on Judaism Emmanuel Levinas,* translated by S. Hand, Maryland: John Hopkins University Press.

Holmes, D. (2001). "From iron gaze to nursing care: Mental health nursing in the era of the panopticism," *Journal of Psychiatric and Mental Health Nursing*, 8(1): 7–15.

Kanvera, A. (2012). "Patient safety in psychiatric inpatient care: A literature review," *Journal of Psychiatric and Mental Health Nursing*, 20(6): 541–548.

Kasmi, Y. (2007). "Characteristics of patients admitted to psychiatric intensive care units," *Irish Journal of Psychological Medicine*, 24(2): 75–78.

Levinas, E. (2006). *Humanism of the Other*, Translated by N. Poller and Introduction by R. A. Cohen, Urbana and Chicago: University of Illinois Press.

Lyon, D. (1994). *The Electronic Eye: The Rise of Surveillance Society*, Minnesota: University of Minnesota Press.

Lyon, D. (2001). *Surveillance and Society: Monitoring Everyday Life*, Buckingham: Open University Press.

Marx, G.T. (1988). *Undercover: Police Surveillance in America*, Berkley: University of California.

Moore, D. (2011) "The benevolent watch: Therapeutic surveillance in drug treatment court," *Theoretical Criminology*, 15(3): 255–268.

Nicki, A. (2001). "The abused mind: Feminist theory, psychiatric disability and trauma," *Hypatia,* 16(4): 80–104.

Norris, C. and Armstrong, G. (1999). *The Maximum Surveillance Society*, London: Routledge.

Rose, N. (1989). *Governing the Soul: The Shaping of the Private Self*, London: Free Association Books.

Simon, B. (2005). "The return of panopticism: Supervision, subjection and the new surveillance," *Surveillance and Society*, 3(1): 1–20.

Soomar, S.M. and Ali, U.U. (2017). "Understanding and managing sexual disinhibition in mentally ill clients," *Psychology and Psychiatry*: Open Access, 1(1): 1–2. Available online: www.omiconline.org/ope-access/understanding-and-managing-sexual-disinhibition-in-mentally-ill-clients-105356.html [accessed 25 September 2019].

Glossary

Asylums Asylums were the historical equivalent of the modern mental health hospital. They were predominantly large Victorian institutions built around city boundaries. Asylums eventually became synonymous with poor treatment of people with mental health disorders. Most patients admitted to asylums did not leave them. Asylums were therefore also known as long-stay hospitals. By the late 1980s, asylums lost favour with the public, resulting in their closure in preference for smaller mental health hospitals.

Forced medication (the "injection") Forced medication involves the administration, with or without seclusion or restraint, of a rapid tranquilliser. The tranquilliser temporarily restricts the patient's freedom of movement. Forced medication is used to control a patient's behaviour in order to reduce risk to their own safety and the safety of other people.

Full-body restraint or restraint It is also known as manual restraint and involves any direct physical contact where the intention is to prevent, restrict or subdue movement of the body (or part of the body) of the patient. Restraint is used to manage a patient's aggressive and disturbed behaviour.

INOP or infrared night-time observation panel This is the use of an infrared CCTV camera placed inside the patient's bedroom, together with audio equipment in order to do night-time nurse observations.

Leave or Section 17 (s.17) Leave Section 17 of the 1983 Mental Health Act (as amended 2007) allows detained patients to be granted leave of absence from the hospital in which they are detained. The aim of this planned leave is to promote the patient's recovery. Only the patient's responsible clinician (RC) is allowed to authorise leave. Any absence from the hospital is regarded as constituting leave. Decisions to allow patients to have leave from the hospital are agreed at weekly multidisciplinary meetings (also known as ward rounds) where the patient's mental health well-being is discussed. Leave can include a short-time off the ward accompanied by one or two staff for a walk around the local area or overnight leave.

Lobotomy Lobotomy, also known as prefrontal leukotomy, is a surgical procedure in which the nerve pathways in a lobe or lobes of the brain are severed. Lobotomies are now referred to as neurosurgery for mental disorder (NMD).

NAPICU National Association of Psychiatric Intensive Care and Low Secure Units

NHS National Health Service

PICU Psychiatric Intensive Care Unit

Post-institutional mental health hospitals The deinstitutionalisation of patient care from large asylums or long-stay hospitals in the late 1970s and 1980s in England and Wales led to the rise of smaller mental health hospitals in the community. Post-institutional mental health hospitals are often integrated with general health care services and community service provision.

Seclusion Seclusion is a method used by mental health staff to manage aggressive and disturbed patients in situations where there is an immediate risk of harm to others. The Mental Health Act Code of Practice (2015, England and Wales) states that seclusion should only take place in a designated seclusion facility that is not used for any other purpose. Seclusion involves removing a patient from the ward environment and placing them in a designated seclusion room. This room is a locked room from which exit is denied.

The Mental Health Act Code of Practice (CoP) 2015 defines Seclusion as "the supervised confinement and isolation of a patient, away from other patients, in an area from which the patient is prevented from leaving, where it is of immediate necessity for the purpose of containment of severe behavioural disturbance which is likely to cause harm to others". (MHA CoP, para 26.103)

Index

For Product Safety Concerns and Information please contact our EU representative GPSR@taylorandfrancis.com
Taylor & Francis Verlag GmbH, Kaufingerstraße 24, 80331 München, Germany

www.ingramcontent.com/pod-product-compliance
Lightning Source LLC
Chambersburg PA
CBHW060311220326
41598CB00027B/4299

* 9 7 8 1 0 3 2 0 1 6 1 1 5 *